Children
for
Health

This book is available from
TALC
PO Box 49
St Albans
Herts AL1 4AX
United Kingdom

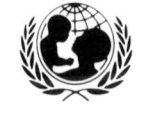

Also distributed
by UNICEF

Cover photograph by John and Penny Hubley

Children for Health

EDITED BY
Hugh Hawes and Christine Scotchmer
with the collaboration of
Audrey Aarons, David Morley & Ella Young

ILLUSTRATED BY
David Gifford

The Child-to-Child Trust
in association with UNICEF

The text of *Children for Health* incorporates all the prime messages contained in *Facts for Life* (UNICEF/WHO/UNESCO/UNFPA, 1993). The supporting information has been slightly shortened. Two new messages have been added.

Additional text has been prepared by a writing team from the Child-to-Child Trust: Audrey Aarons, Hugh Hawes, David Morley, Christine Scotchmer and Ella Young.

You are welcome to adapt, translate and modify any part or parts of the text of this book without requesting permission from the authors or publishers. The materials, including the illustrations, are all copyright-free and we hope that you will use them whenever you need to. We should be grateful, however, if you could let us see a copy of your work.

Photographs used as artist's references for illustrations:
By John Hubley for page 72
By Caroline Penn/OXFAM for page 86
By Caroline Penn/IPPF for page 152
By UNICEF for page 172

© Child-to-Child Trust

First published 1993

British Library Cataloguing-in-Publication Data
Children for Health
I. Hawes, Hugh II. Scotchmer, Christine
613.0432091724

ISBN 0-946182-05-1

Designed by John C. Wright
Typeset by Domino Typesetting & Origination
Printed by Werner Söderström Oy

Contents

PART ONE

Children as Partners

Children for Health	9
Facts for Life	10
Helping Children to Help Others	13
Three Levels of Action	19
Who Benefits?	30
Ideas into Action	32
Evaluation	36

PART TWO

Health Messages and Children's Action

Twelve Messages to Save and Improve Lives	46
Breastfeeding	48
Child Growth	60
Child Development	72
Hygiene	86
Diarrhoea	100
Immunization	114
Coughs and Colds	124
Malaria	134
AIDS	142
Safe Motherhood	152
Accidents	162
Food for the Family	172
Some Useful Resources	182

Children for Health has been produced by the Child-to-Child Trust, with financial assistance from UNICEF and MISEREOR. The Trust is based at the Institutes of Education and Child Health of the University of London.

A parallel publication, *Les Enfants pour la Santé*, has been prepared in Paris by a team from L'Enfant pour l'Enfant under the direction of Elisabeth Dumurgier. L'Enfant pour l'Enfant is based at the Institute of Health and Development of the University of Paris. Both teams have consulted frequently and exchanged ideas during the course of writing.

The Child-to-Child Trust thanks all those who have read and commented on the manuscript; and is grateful to the Save the Children Fund (UK) for financing the participation of Audrey Aarons in the initial writing workshop.

The Child-to-Child Trustees dedicate this book to the memory of Beverley Young who, as much as any other single individual, has influenced the philosophy of the movement and the spread of its ideas worldwide.

Facts for Life & Children for Health

Since its first publication in 1989, *Facts for Life* has met with a worldwide response. Over 100 countries have produced translations or adaptations and a total of some eight million copies in over 170 languages are currently in use.

The appeal of *Facts for Life* is simple. There is a broad agreement among medical experts on the essential child health information that all families have a right to know. *Facts for Life* brings that information together. It is the most authoritative expression, in plain language, of what medical science now knows about practical, low-cost ways of protecting children's lives and health.

- It is information which can help to save the lives of many millions of children in the developing world.
- It is information which can significantly reduce malnutrition and help to protect the healthy growth of the next generation.
- It is information which almost all parents can put into practice, in some degree, at very low cost.

Facts for Life is published by UNICEF, WHO, UNESCO, and UNFPA, in partnership with over 160 of the world's best-known children's agencies.

The revised edition of *Facts for Life* takes into account the many comments received from users over the last four years and has been thoroughly reviewed in the light of the most recent research in the various fields covered (including AIDS).

In response to requests from many countries, a new chapter has been added on the mental and emotional development of children.

Communicators

Every week, a quarter of a million children die in the developing world. Many millions more live on with ill health and poor growth.

A fundamental cause of this tragedy is poverty. Another fundamental cause is that today's knowledge about protecting the health and growth of children has not yet been put at the disposal of the majority.

Facts for Life helps to make this knowledge more widely available.

But experience has shown that only frequent repetition of new information, from many trusted sources and over many years, can truly succeed in putting new health information at the disposal of all families and communities.

Facts for Life is issued as a long-term communication challenge to:

- Heads of state and political leaders
- Educational systems and the teaching profession
- The medical profession and the health services
- Media professionals in television and radio, newspapers and magazines
- Religious and spiritual leaders
- Employers and the business community
- Trade union and co-operative leaders
- Community health workers, nurses, and midwives
- Development workers and voluntary agencies
- Women's organizations
- Youth movements
- Community organizations and traditional leaders
- All departments of national and local government
- Artists, writers, entertainers, sportsmen and -women

In sum, *Facts for Life* is for all those who can help to undertake the greatests communications challenge of all – the challenge of empowering families to use today's knowledge to protect today's children – and tomorrow's world.

Children for Health, which includes all the messages contained in the latest edition of *Facts for Life*, is designed for those who work with children and who believe that children, in schools and as family members, need to be considered as partners in spreading health messages as well as benefiting from them. We support this belief, and welcome children as communicators of *Facts for Life*.

James P Grant
Executive Director
United Nations Children's Fund
(UNICEF)

Dr Hiroshi Nakajima
Director-General
World Health Organization
(WHO)

Federico Mayor
Director-General
United Nations Educational, Scientific, and Cultural Organization
(UNESCO)

Dr Nafis Sadik
Executive Director
The United Nations Population Fund
(UNFPA)

PART ONE
Children as Partners

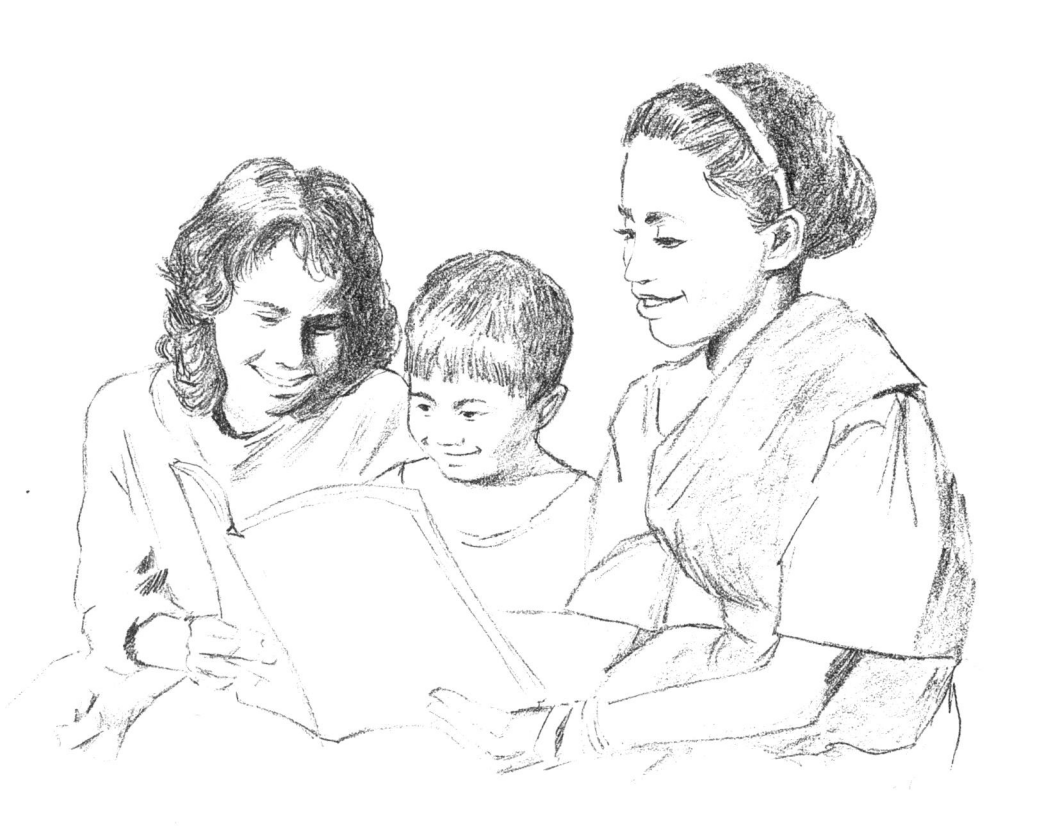

We Know a Child

'We know somebody who is a teacher and a health worker. She looks after two children. One is four and one is two. She keeps them safe. She carries the little one and picks him up when he cries. She protects the bigger one from accidents. Yesterday when the little girl went too near the stove she scolded her. Today she helped her to cross the road and taught her how to watch for the cars.

She helps them when they are sick. She makes them comfortable, brings them food and keeps the flies away. Last month she saved the life of the little boy. He had diarrhoea and was very weak but she sat near him and gave him water through the day and long into the night. The little boy lived. Early in the year before the rains she noticed that the bigger girl had a sore on her leg. She took the girl to the medical post and the sore was cured.

She helps them to grow healthy. She feeds the little boy when he is hungry; she helps the little girl find sticks to clean her teeth. She teaches her songs to help her remember good health habits. She plays with the boy and she plays with the girl. As they play they learn to use their hands and bodies to try out things, to think of things, to imagine things. This teacher makes toys for them, invents games for them and tells stories to them. She teaches them words and how to sew words together.

Who is this teacher who does so much for her pupils and does it so well? She is their elder sister – and she is eleven years old.

We know a group of community workers who know every inch of the village in which they work, who are accepted by everyone, who want to help their community, who will work hard (for short periods of time) and cheerfully (all the time). Last month the health worker used them to collect information about which children had been vaccinated in the village. Next Tuesday some of them will help to remind the villagers that the baby clinic is coming and they will be at hand to play with the older children when mothers take their babies to see the nurse. Next month they plan to help the schoolteacher in a village clean-up campaign. These health workers are the boys and girls of the village.' *

---

* Aarons, A, Hawes, H and Gayton, J (1979). *CHILD-to-child*. London: Macmillan.

CHILDREN FOR HEALTH

This is a book for those who work with and for children. It is based on the belief that children not only need to *have* better health but are also able to *give* better health to others. We who work with children must help them to do so. Who are 'we'?

We are all those who plan programmes, write materials, train teachers and health workers and who work with children and their families in schools and communities. This is a book for all of us. It is not a text for children; not a lesson by lesson guide for teachers. It is a resource book of ideas. We can use them in many different ways.

Policy makers can use them in planning. We hope that they will decide that the messages should be learnt by all children, who should be enabled and encouraged to act on them and pass them on.

Curriculum planners can use them. We hope they will introduce them into national programmes for schools; integrate them into subject syllabuses and into textbooks; and recommend methodologies which promote children's active involvement.

Health education planners can adopt them and introduce them into their programmes both in schools and with non-school-going children.

Teacher trainers can use them. We hope they will introduce them into the programmes of *teachers' colleges* so that all teachers-to-be know the facts and how to help children act on them, and into *in-service* programmes so that serving teachers can become aware of them.

Schools can use them as a resource: the ideas in this book will help *heads* to plan school-based health programmes and activities, *teachers* to introduce activities into their lessons, and *children* to take ideas back to their families.

Clubs and youth groups based on the school will find these ideas particularly valuable.

Organizers of *out-of-school groups* can also use this book since none of the activities it contains are necessarily classroom-based.

1. Facts for Life

Health action is based upon sound health knowledge. Before we *act* we need to *know* essential facts. The book *Facts for Life* was first published in 1989, jointly by UNICEF, UNESCO and the World Health Organization. It contains 10 sections, each setting out essential survival and development messages. In their preliminary statement to *Facts for Life* the directors of the three agencies describe the messages in these terms:

'Today, there is a world-wide scientific consensus on essential child health information.

● It is information which can help to save the lives of many millions of children in the world.

● It is information which can drastically reduce malnutrition and help to protect the healthy growth of the next generation.

● It is information which almost all parents can put into practice, in some degree, at very low cost.

It is therefore information to which all families now have a right.'

Facts for Life **was revised in 1993. The 'facts' are divided into 11 sections:**

- **Timing Births**
- **Safe Motherhood**
- **Breastfeeding**
- **Child Growth**
- **Immunization**
- **Diarrhoea**
- **Coughs and Colds**
- **Hygiene**
- **Malaria**
- **AIDS**
- **Child Development**

Each section begins with the words 'What every family and community has a right to know about ...' and includes a small number of prime messages and supporting information.

In *Children for Health* we include the complete text of the prime messages and all the supporting information in seven of the 11 sections, though we have changed their order. We have slightly shortened Breastfeeding, Timing Births and Safe Motherhood, and combined Safe Motherhood and Timing Births in one section. We have added prime messages and supporting information on Nursing Children with Fever to the section on Malaria.

We have included two additional sections because they are vital for children to know about and very rich in activities which children can do. These sections are Accidents and Food for the Family.

Our 12 sections in their new order are, therefore:

- **Breastfeeding**
- **Child Growth**
- **Child Development**
- **Hygiene**
- **Diarrhoea**
- **Immunization**
- **Coughs and Colds**
- **Malaria**
- **AIDS**
- **Safe Motherhood**
- **Accidents**
- **Food for the Family**

By mid-1993 eight million copies of *Facts for Life* had been sold in 178 languages. Leading medical personnel from all round the world gave their expertise free in the drafting, checking and revision of the work. 165 organizations have been enrolled as partners in communicating the messages.

A companion book *Using Facts for Life – A Handbook* draws on worldwide experience to suggest how the information in *Facts for Life* can be put into practice effectively at local level.

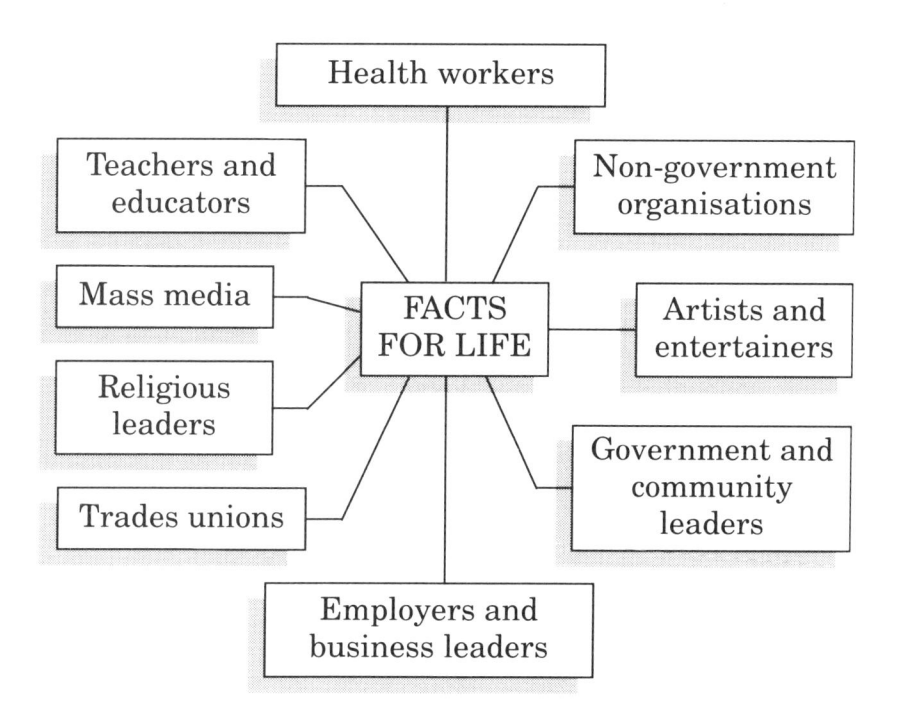

```
                    ┌─────────────────┐
                    │  Health workers │
                    └─────────────────┘
    ┌──────────────┐                    ┌──────────────────┐
    │ Teachers and │                    │  Non-government  │
    │  educators   │                    │  organisations   │
    └──────────────┘                    └──────────────────┘
    ┌──────────────┐   ┌───────────┐    ┌──────────────────┐
    │  Mass media  │───│ FACTS     │    │  Artists and     │
    └──────────────┘   │ FOR LIFE  │    │  entertainers    │
    ┌──────────────┐   └───────────┘    └──────────────────┘
    │  Religious   │                    ┌──────────────────┐
    │   leaders    │                    │ Government and   │
    └──────────────┘                    │   community      │
    ┌──────────────┐                    │    leaders       │
    │Trades unions │                    └──────────────────┘
    └──────────────┘
                  ┌────────────────────┐
                  │   Employers and    │
                  │  business leaders  │
                  └────────────────────┘
```

11

Women's education

At the beginning of *Facts for Life* the following important words occur:

> 'Putting today's essential health knowledge into practice will be seen by many as "women's work".
>
> ... the greatest communication challenge of all is the challenge of communicating the idea that the time has come, in all countries, for men to share more fully in that most difficult and important of all responsibilities – protecting the lives and the health and the growth of their children.
>
> *Facts for Life* is therefore addressed not only to women but to men.'

There is more to say:
In many countries, boys still have more schooling, better nutrition and health care, and more opportunities in life than girls. Yet both have the same rights as individuals to all of these, and equal responsibilities as parents. Research has proved that women who are better educated are healthier and bring up healthier children who achieve better in education and life. Hence women's education is not only their birthright but is directly linked to the health and success of future communities.

Facts for Life and the World Summit for Children

In the declaration signed by heads of state at the World Summit for Children in 1990, the world's leaders committed themselves to a 10 point programme to protect the rights of the child and improve children's lives. The 10 points include enhancing children's health; promoting optimal growth and development in childhood; strengthening the role of women and respecting the role of the family – all issues which are addressed in *Facts for Life*.

The declaration ends with a plea for partnership to meet the challenge, and contains the following statement:

> 'Among the partnerships we seek, we turn especially to children themselves. We appeal to them to participate in this effort.' *

This book is a response to this appeal.

---

*World Summit for Children (1990). *World Declaration on the Survival, Protection and Development of Children*. New York: United Nations.

Facts for Life and Education for All

In 1990 the *World Declaration on Education for All* was issued in Jomtien, Thailand. The declaration emphasizes the right of all citizens to basic education and discusses how this may be provided. Basic education is not to be defined as so many years spent in school or ground covered by an official syllabus. Rather it focuses on learning and skills attained, whether in school or outside it, whether by children, youth or even adults. Such basic learning skills are necessary for further learning and help learners to acquire what has been described as a 'driving permit for life'.

Article 1 of the Declaration reads:

> '*Every person – child, youth and adult – shall be able to benefit from educational opportunities designed to meet their basic learning needs.* These needs comprise both essential learning tools (such as literacy, oral expression, numeracy, and problem solving) and the basic learning content (such as knowledge, skills, values, and attitudes) required by human beings to be able to survive, to develop their full capacities, to live and work in dignity, to participate fully in development, to improve the quality of their lives, to make informed decisions, and to continue learning.' *

All governments would agree that health content and health skills are vital to enable human beings to survive, to participate fully and to improve the quality of their lives and that health education should enable them to make informed decisions. What is less certain is how to define and select this content and these skills. This book helps us to do so.

2. Helping Children to Help Others

What do we mean by 'health'?

We all hope and pray for our children to grow up healthy and happy. We wish them to live a productive and stimulating life. We expect them to have rights as citizens, to live in peace, to live in an environment which has been preserved from contamination and exploitation.

We are also aware that for many world citizens these hopes are not fulfilled – that millions of children die as infants, that many who survive are weakened by hunger and disease, and that

---

*Inter-Agency Commission for the World Conference on Education For All (1990). *World Declaration on Education For All*. New York: UNICEF.

many grow up in societies and environments which are not as we would want them to be.

Individuals may feel powerless to change the future for their children or to shape the society in which these children will grow up, but all individuals have some degree of control over their family's health and well-being and when individuals are 'all for health' they can all make a big difference.

Being healthy starts with being alive, thus the world's emphasis on *child survival*; but we quickly pass beyond survival to *development*, beyond simple ideas of health as 'not being ill' to wider ideas of health as physical, mental, emotional and social health. Thus, the World Health Organization has defined health as:

'A state of complete physical, mental and social well-being and not merely the absence of disease.'

Moreover, we need to recognize that human beings live on a planet and have the responsibility to preserve its resources for future generations. Currently many of us, starting with industrialized nations, are plundering and destroying these resources. Our own health depends on the health of the environment:

If we destroy the soil, we starve.

If we pollute the water, we sicken.

If we infect the air we breathe, we die.

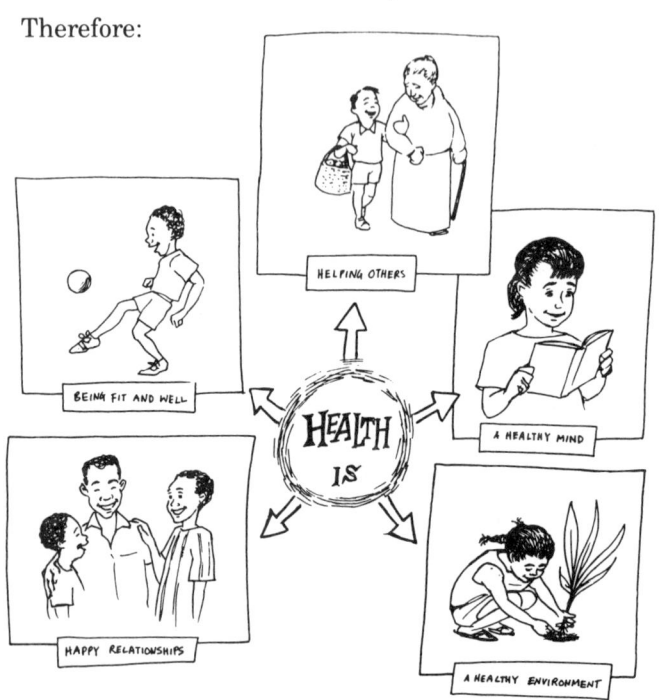

Therefore:

Health is everyone's concern

Every individual has a right to basic health knowledge and health care but also a duty to help others maintain and improve their health. The health of a community depends to a very great degree upon whether its citizens are passive or active towards health.

Passive citizens wait for others to provide better health for them.

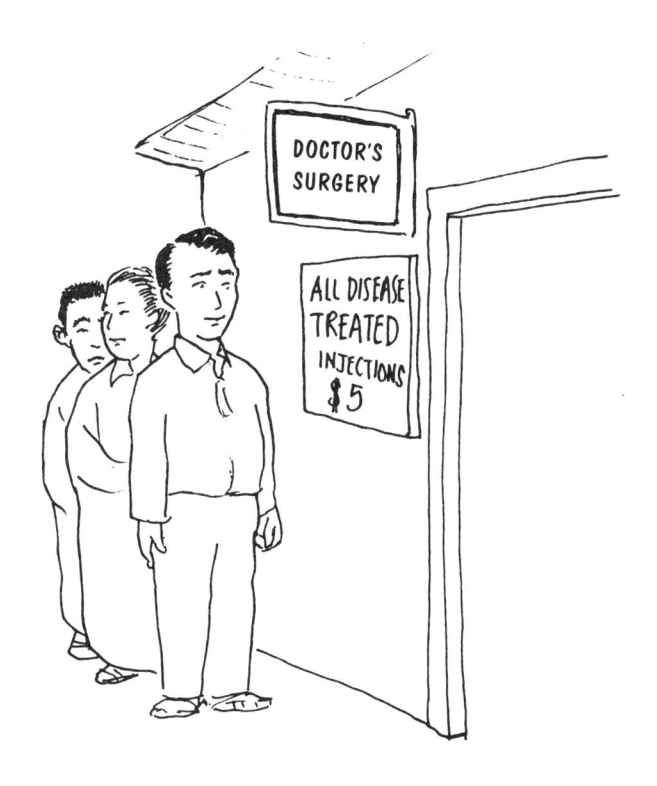

Active citizens promote better health for others through:

- Keeping themselves healthy.
- Taking action to *prevent* disease and distress in their families and communities.
- Treating conditions which they can treat themselves and recognizing those which they cannot.
- Taking action to improve their neighbourhood environment.
- Passing on their knowledge to those who do not have it.
- Giving help to others who need it.

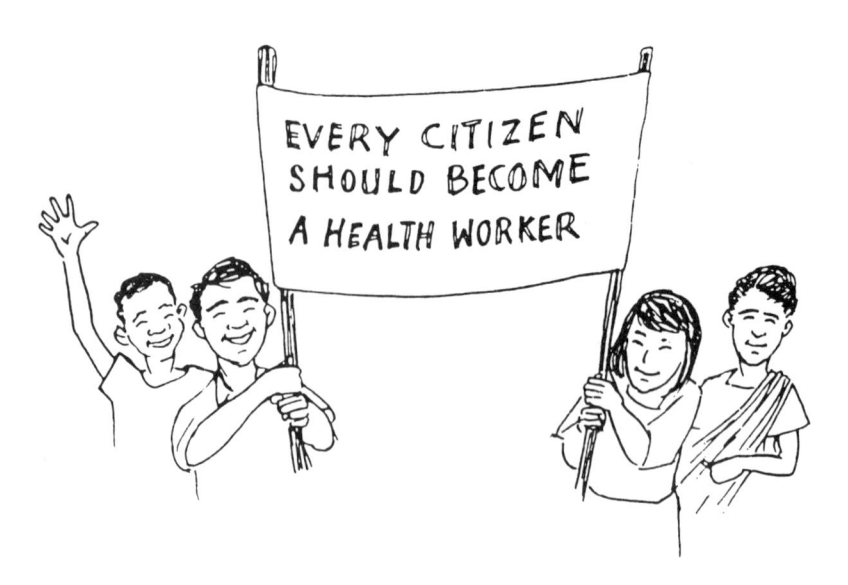

Children as partners in promoting healthy living

Strength, effectiveness and happiness in communities often come from the strength, love and co-operation of the families who live in them.

The definition of a family as mother, father and children may often prove too restrictive. Grandparents, other relatives, friends and neighbours can all take family responsibility for children and provide the love, security and sense of solidarity they need. But some children are denied adult support; these children, brought up in institutions, living on the streets, exploited in the work place, have only their own comradeship to fall back on for support.

All children are citizens, those with the benefit of family support and those without it. In many countries nearly half the citizens are below 15 years old. Just as adult citizens have rights and duties towards health, so do children.

Child citizens can promote better health by:

- Keeping healthy and setting a good example – Amina cleans her teeth.

- Preventing disease and distress – Musa covers the water pot; comforts his little sister.

- Treating conditions which they can, and recognizing those they cannot – Sunil cleans her little brother's nose when he has a cold; calls in her parents when he has a fever and is breathing too fast.

- Taking action to improve their neighbourhood – Pedro and Anna build a fence round the well.
- Passing on their knowledge to others – Class 5 in school show a play about the dangers of bottle-feeding.
- Giving help to others who need it – Patrick holds Mary's hand crossing the road.

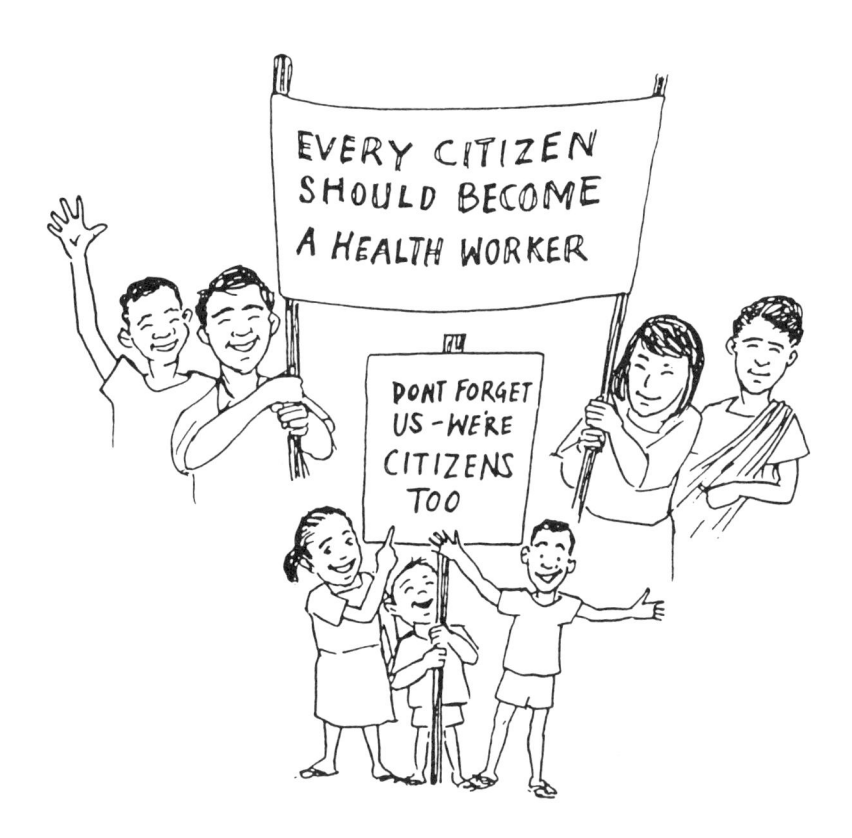

All children are health workers, boys as well as girls.

    Boys can   Look after babies
                             Cook good food
                             Nurse children while they are sick
                             just as well as girls can
    Girls can   Keep our neighbourhood clean
                             Practise first aid
                             Carry out immunization surveys
                             just as well as boys can

When children become partners in promoting health they contribute something special to the partnership. Children have special advantages and special roles in spreading health to others.

Younger children often spend more time with older children than with adults. They admire them, copy them and do what they say.

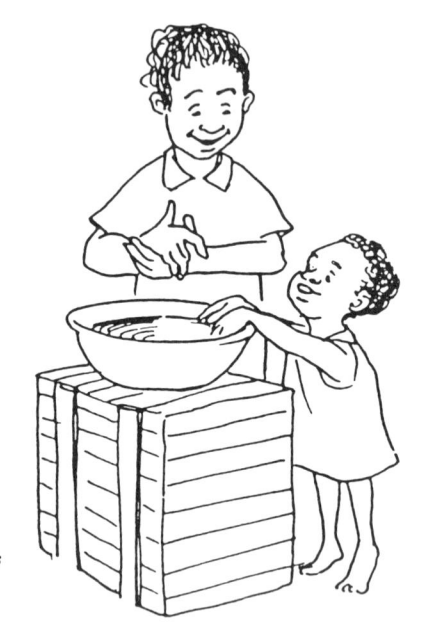

Washing my hands like my sister

Groups of children, particularly influential and popular groups, can influence their peers in a way which adults can never do.

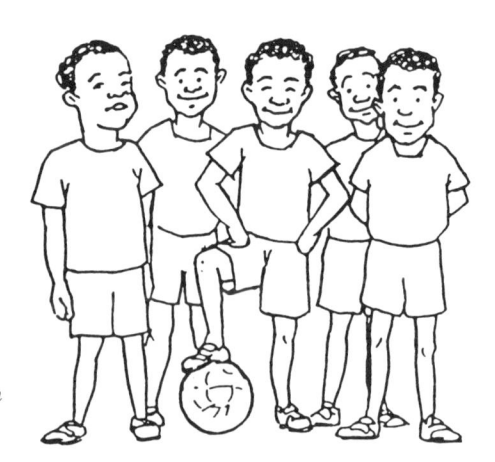

The football team doesn't smoke

Children, through their innocence, can often remind adults that their actions are unwise or unsafe. They can act as the conscience of a community.

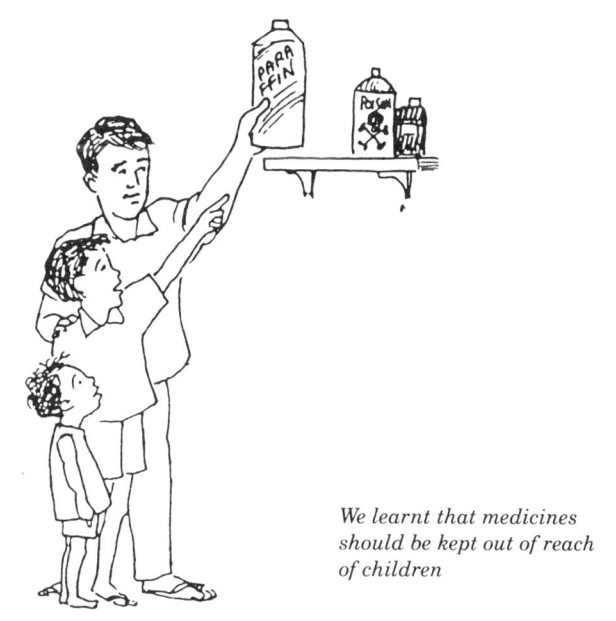

We learnt that medicines should be kept out of reach of children

3. Three Levels of Action

Children cannot start and maintain programmes on their own. They need support from adults; from teachers, health workers, youth leaders and community members.

Teachers and youth leaders also need support from those who plan programmes and provide materials.

Thus there are three levels of action:

Programme organizers to teachers and community workers.
Teachers and community workers to children.
Children to other children, families and communities.

Action from programme organizers

Programme organizers need to:

- Choose messages and action that are most suitable for children to take up.

    Activities need to be:
    ☐ Important for community health.
    ☐ Appropriate and do-able by children.
    ☐ Interesting and fun to do.

- Define and explain general objectives for the programme and its activities.

    Objectives should be:
    - Clear and medically accurate.
    - In line with other programmes and priorities (so that children's action can reinforce other health action).
    - Achievable.

- Train field workers.

    Field workers need to:
    - Have correct medical and scientific knowledge and keep it up-to-date.
    - Acquire confidence to adapt national programmes to local needs.
    - Encourage active methods for children to understand and act on.
    - Develop skills to listen to people's concerns, understand their needs, and adapt national programmes to meet these needs.
    - Learn how to monitor activities.

- Help in production and adaptation of materials.

    Materials need to be:
    - Appropriate to local needs and cultures.
    - Medically accurate.
    - Easily readable.
    - Interesting and fun to work with.

Remember: All these tasks require time and expertise. Programme organizers need support and assistance from policy makers, professional bodies, NGOs, the local business communities and international agencies.

Action from teachers, health workers and youth leaders

These work directly with children who need their knowledge, guidance and encouragement to be effective.

Four steps for planning and action

Many field programmes find a four step methodology a useful approach to planning and organizing children's action.

Recognize and Understand ... Study ... Act ... Evaluate

Project workers in Mexico draw a bus with four wheels to help explain this methodology.

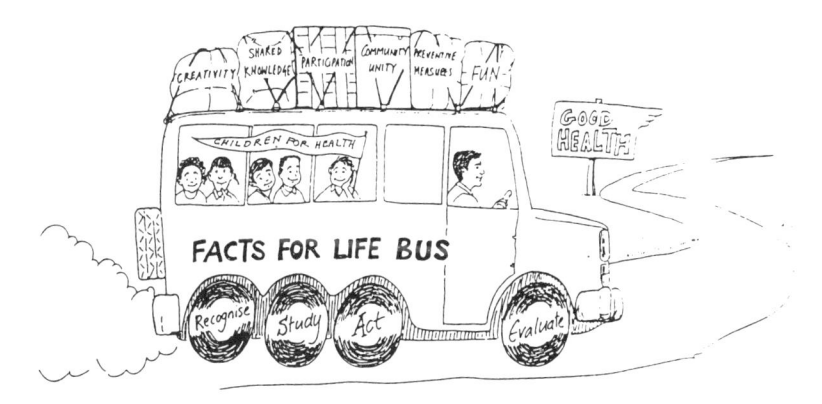

Thus children need to:

Step 1
- **Recognize** health needs and priorities e.g. Diarrhoea kills babies.
- **Understand** the main message e.g. What causes diarrhoea; what dehydration is; why it kills; how we can prevent it.

Step 2
- **Study:**
    - ☐ **Find out more** e.g. A survey: diarrhoea in our families (how many children have had it? were they breastfed or bottle-fed? how is it treated?).
    - ☐ **Discuss findings** e.g. Which local treatments are helpful or may be harmful?
    - ☐ **Learn skills** e.g. Recognizing dehydration; making a rehydration drink.

Step 3
- **Act:**
    - ☐ **Plan action** e.g. What can I do? What can we do (children together)? Who can help us?
    - ☐ **Take action myself** e.g. Help baby to drink.
    - ☐ **Take action with others** e.g. Make a puppet show.

Step 4
- **Evaluate:**
    - ☐ **Discuss action taken** e.g. What did we do? Who listened to us? What improved? What didn't?
    - ☐ **Plan new action** e.g. Let's discuss with our teachers and the health worker what most needs doing next.

Active approaches to learning and teaching health

Sound knowledge and understanding are the basis of effective action for health. School work leading towards examinations does not always promote understanding and rarely encourages action.

Sometimes schools talk of 'active learning' and 'active methods'. Activity on its own does not achieve learning. What is needed are methods which promote active and critical thinking, leading to well-planned and effective action.

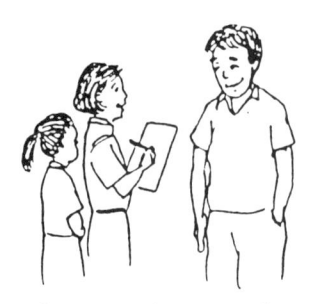

METHODS WHICH PROMOTE UNDERSTANDING

Surveys in the community   *Discussing together*   *Practical activities*

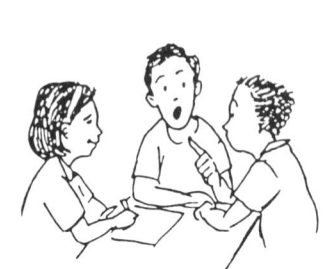

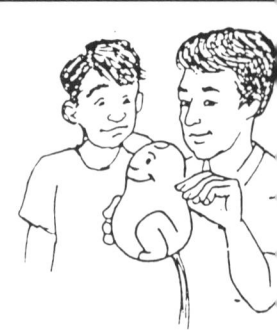

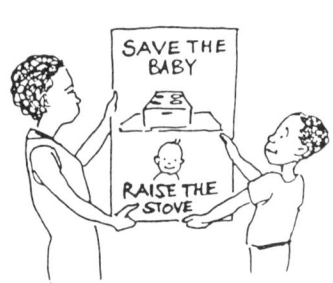

METHODS WHICH HELP CHILDREN COMMUNICATE MESSAGES

Campaigns, school fairs and open days   *Picture- and poster-making*

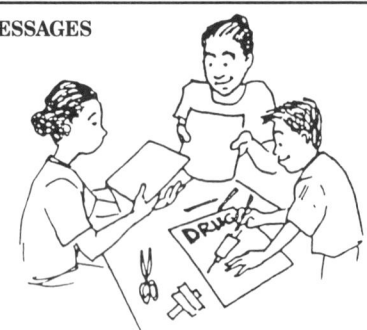

METHODS WHICH HELP CHILDREN TO EVALUATE THE EFFECT OF THEIR ACTIONS

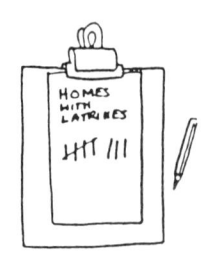

Observing and recording   *Describing*   *Measuring*

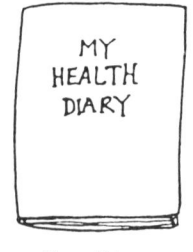

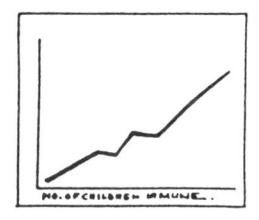

Remember: These new approaches to sound planning and active learning take time. Teachers and others who help children need support from doctors and health workers who give authority to their messages; from their employers and inspectors who can encourage and praise their work and provide any available resources; and from the community to encourage and assist them.

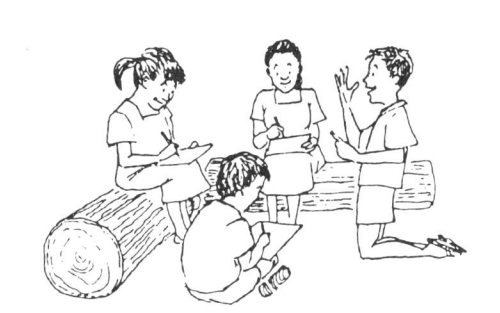

Story-telling/story-writing with discussion

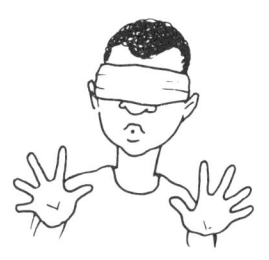

Role-playing

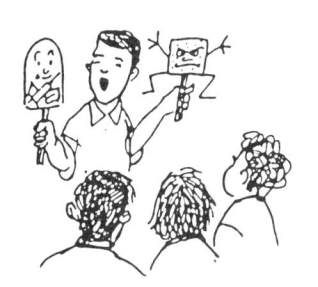

Drama and puppets

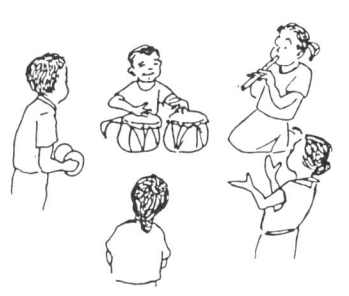

Songs and dances

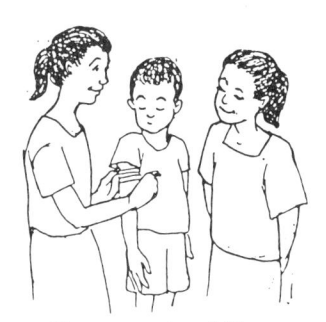

Demonstrating skills

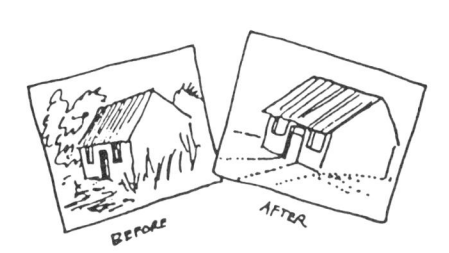

Comparing

Action from children to other children, their families and their communities

Children can spread messages and take action in different places:

- **At school** they can:
    - ☐ Learn together actively.
    - ☐ Help and teach their friends.
    - ☐ Help and protect younger children.
    - ☐ Help make the school surroundings clean and healthy.

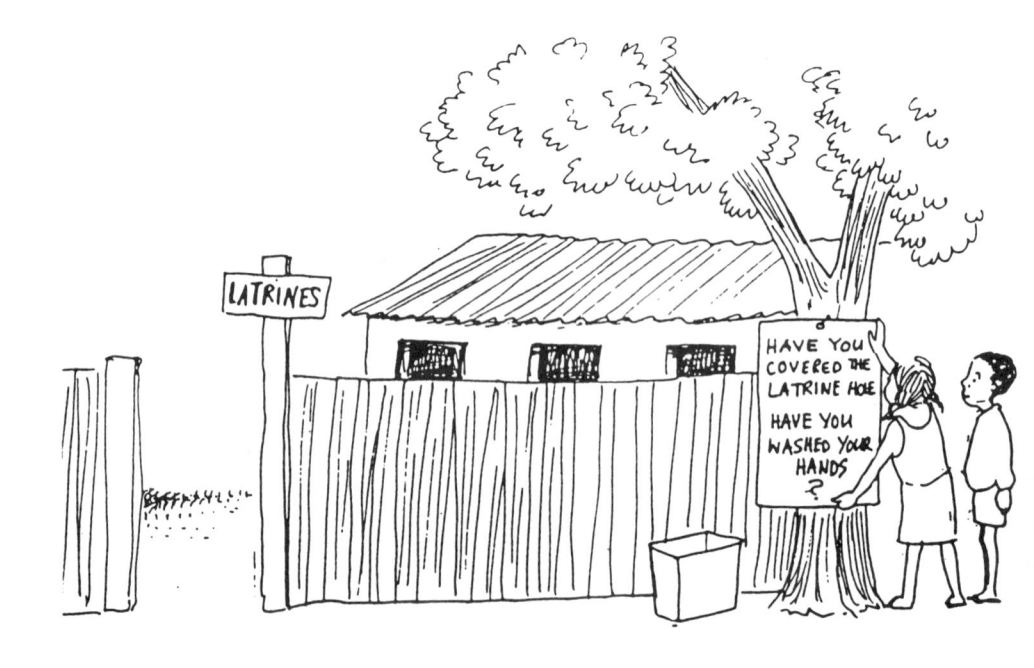

- **At home** they can:
    - ☐ Describe and demonstrate what they have learnt at school.
    - ☐ Help their families in good health practices.
    - ☐ Teach and help younger brothers and sisters.
    - ☐ Play with and help other children who have not gone to school.

□ Keep the home surroundings clean and safe.

□ Reinforce health messages received through mass media such as radio.

- **In the community** they can:

    □ Pass on messages through plays and songs (often during campaigns organized by the school or the health worker).

    □ Act as messengers and helpers for the health worker (e.g. reminding families about immunization).

    □ Participate in health action in the community.

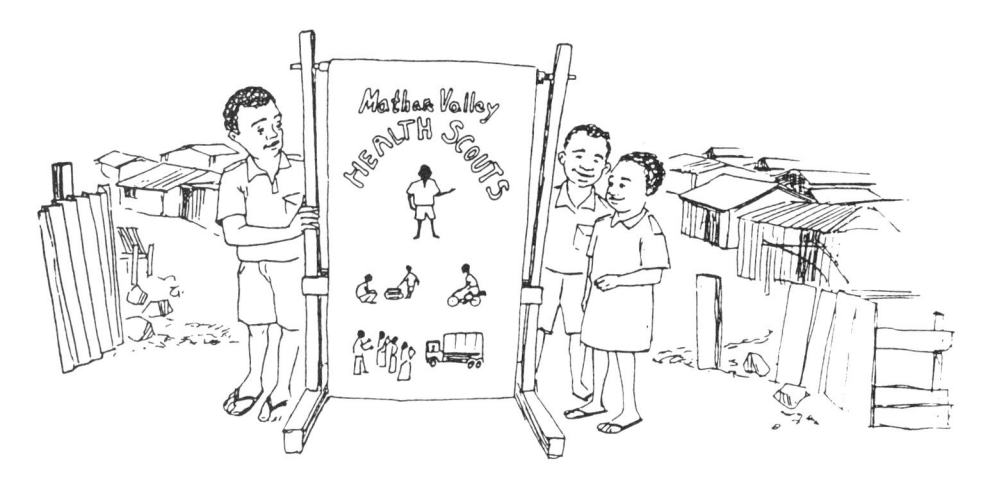

Children can spread messages either singly or together:

□ Often one child communicates best with another child; older to younger, friend to friend; schoolchild to out-of-school child. Sometimes a child can tell something she has learnt in school to her father or mother and they will find it useful. Sometimes she can set an example which others in the family will copy (e.g. making a picture book and showing it to baby).

□ Sometimes two children can give support to each other (e.g. making a survey together; explaining health messages to older children; helping a child with learning difficulties).

□ Often older children can work together, particularly when they are passing on messages through plays and songs to adults. Each of our 12 sections contains activities which one child can do, as well as others which are better done by children together.

Children's action singly or together

THE MESSAGE	ONE CHILD	CHILDREN WORKING TOGETHER
Breastfeeding	...helps her young sister while mother is breastfeeding	...perform a play about the dangers of bottle-feeding
Child Growth	...helps mother fill in a 'road to health' chart	...survey eating patterns in the community
Child Development	...makes a mobile for baby	...hold a toy workshop
Hygiene	...cleans fingernails of a younger child at school	...make and use water pots and ladles
Diarrhoea	...makes a rehydration drink out of rice water	...demonstrate dehydration to other children using a 'gourd baby'
Immunization	...makes a birthday card for baby (with immunization schedule)	...participate in an immunization campaign planned by the health worker
Coughs and Colds	...feeds a brother who has a cold	...demonstrate signs of pneumonia to a parents' meeting
Malaria	...retells a story, 'The Lion's Fever', he has read at school	...destroy mosquito larvae
AIDS	...helps someone with AIDS	...write and perform a play about AIDS
Safe Motherhood	...helps mother when she is pregnant	...hold a puppet show to demonstrate how children born too close together can suffer ill health
Accidents	...takes responsibility for younger child crossing the road	...make a survey of safety of medicines at home
Food for the Family	...helps a younger child to plant vegetables at home	...plant trees to conserve soil

Remember: Being 'health workers' is not easy for children, even though they enjoy doing it. Sometimes they are unsure of themselves, sometimes they are nervous, sometimes they can lose heart or lose interest. They need support, advice, praise and encouragement from us all. Within their own cultures they may encounter resistance to their role, and may have to find their own special means of communicating ideas in a way which is acceptable to adults.

Is it easy?

At all levels those who introduce *Facts for Life* and encourage children to act upon them will meet difficulties. Questions will be asked and doubts expressed.

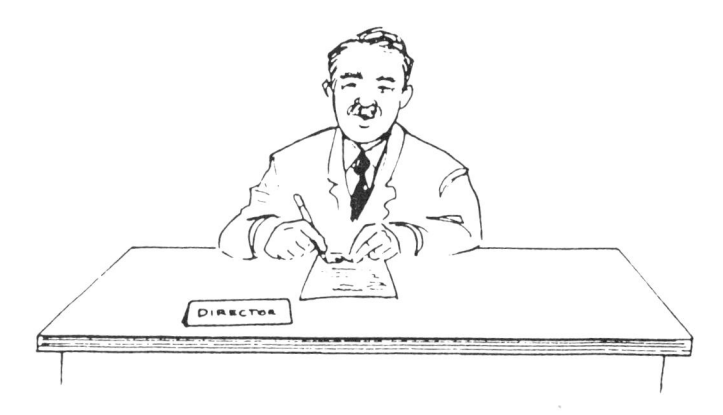

The policy maker asks:

'What's this new approach? Is it worthwhile?'

'Where are the resources to launch it? Which ministry will be in charge?'

Some responses:

'In many ways the approach is not new. We have always valued children and put other children in their trust. This approach confirms our trust and provides new knowledge and new opportunities for children to learn to be better parents and community members.'

'Apart from training, involving children does not imply extra resources. Indeed, children represent one of the resources which every nation has.'

'Good health depends on co-operation *between* sectors. Whenever education and health have co-operated effectively both have benefited.'

The school head and youth group organizer ask:

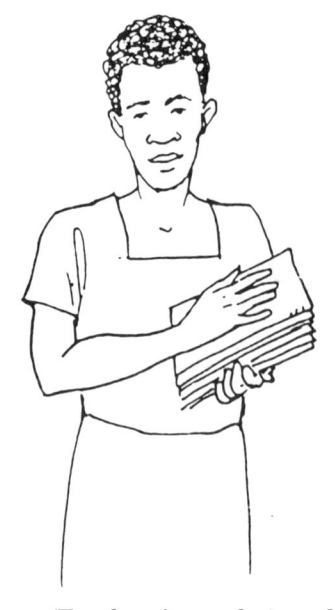

'What's new about this? We always do it. It's called hygiene teaching.'

'Our programme is overcrowded. We have examinations. Is there a place to fit this in?'

'Teachers' morale is so low. Will they take it on?'

'How can we attempt it when we have so few materials?'

Some responses:

'The approach is *not* just conventional hygiene teaching, and must not be allowed to become so. By activating and consulting children they become interested and involved in a way they never did before.'

'The approach does not imply new subjects and new teaching. It fits easily into existing subjects such as science, language and mathematics (think of weighing and measuring, and making graphs). Much activity can take place in clubs and groups after school time. Examination questions in other subjects *can* include health content – but knowledge about keeping alive and healthy is well worth acquiring for its own sake.'

'Teachers, even unpaid and undervalued, are naturally interested in health topics. They must survive too. They become more interested when they see children's enthusiasm.'

'Field programmes do face grievous constraints. Fortunately many health approaches such as discussions, songs, drama and child stimulation can be achieved with no resources except enthusiasm.'

The parent asks:

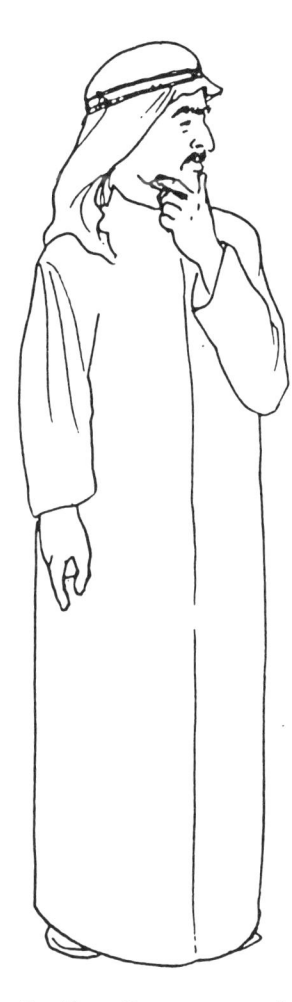

'Are these new ideas undermining our customs and beliefs?'

'Should children be teaching others instead of learning from their elders?'

Some responses:

'Many customs and beliefs, far from being questioned need to be reinforced and strengthened through these approaches. And as for the others ... people are changing. Younger, better educated mothers and fathers are now prepared to question practices which cause deaths of infants, which give girls less life chances than boys, or which discriminate against the weak and the sick. When schools teach children that these customs are dangerous many mothers and fathers will welcome such teaching.'

'Any practice or approach which lessens the respect of children for their families should be discouraged. But as we have indicated there are many ways in which children can work *with families* for change. This book suggests many ideas all of which have been proved effective in societies round the world.'

4. Who Benefits?

At first sight it may seem that we are looking at children as agents for providing health to *target groups* (other children, families and communities). The most important thing therefore is to find out whether the message 'shot' by the child 'hit' that target.

However once we begin to think of children as *partners* in a much more complicated process – *changing lives* rather than hitting targets – we can see that many more benefits result.

Children benefit

The children who pass on the messages learn and understand more, develop confidence and a sense of self-worth, develop awareness of the needs of others and good social attitudes to them. They also develop communication skills because they must pass on their ideas to others.

I FEEL IMPORTANT THEY LISTENED TO ME

The children who are helped by others may understand better because another child is explaining to them. In some programmes a special attempt is made to identify children who may lack helpers and friends (especially children who are disabled or in distress). For these the assistance and companionship of another child can be sunlight in their lives.

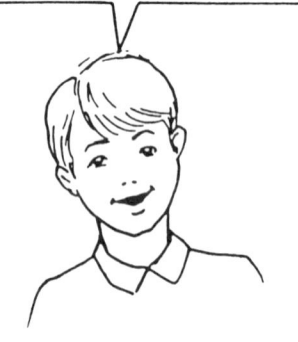

All children gain from participation in a health programme which links learning with action. They will remember what they have done when the words in the textbooks and upon the blackboard are long forgotten.

Moreover, children have health needs which can be met here and now. Through their knowledge and actions they can increase their chances of remaining healthy and happy – tomorrow, next week, next month, as well as over the longer term when they become parents themselves.

Schools benefit

Schools can benefit from more interesting and more effective teaching and learning methods. They can use these to develop knowledge and learning skills which children can relate to their needs and their 'world'.

Evidence is now growing that when a school is involved in a successful Child-to-Child and Child-to-Community programme, children in the programme are more likely to attend regularly and do better in class.

Schools also benefit from closer links with the community and its needs, and with health workers and health services within that community.

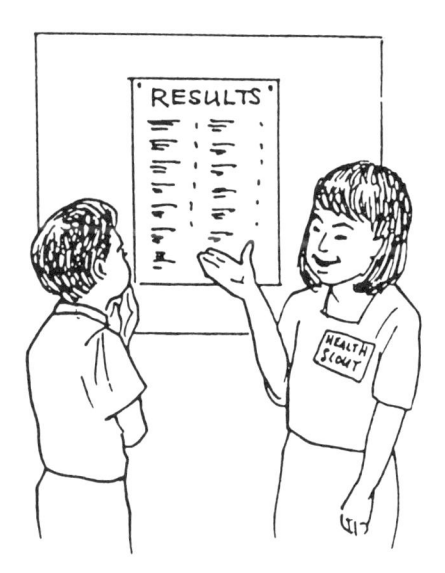

Families and communities benefit

Very real, sometimes dramatic, health gains are possible when children are mobilized to spread messages. In programmes such as control of scabies, child campaigns have been known almost to eliminate the condition. When there is a local campaign, e.g. on immunization, children's participation can greatly strengthen it.

When schools, children, youth are jointly involved alongside health workers, communities can be fully united in a movement towards Health for All.

When children are seen as knowledgeable and concerned in the health of a family it strengthens that family and increases the mutual respect which is so vital in promoting the rights of the child.

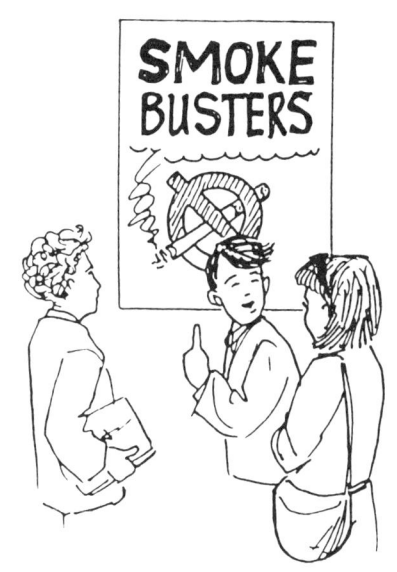

5. Ideas into Action

This section suggests ways of starting, building and maintaining programmes which help children to communicate *Facts for Life* messages and take action based on them. These suggestions are based on worldwide experience gained from Child-to-Child and related programmes. Such experience suggests that although co-operation is vital between all sectors, especially health and education at national, regional and local levels, it is *education* which may be best suited to take the lead in planning and co-ordinating activities.

Getting started

1. A national consensus

Improvements in health are measured in actions rather than words. Nevertheless statements of intent are important. Once there is a national agreement that as a component of their basic education *every child (as part of a family) has a right to know Facts for Life and should be encouraged to pass on and act upon that knowledge*, then all those who are already undertaking activities or who wish to start them will be enabled and encouraged.

2. Success stories and sharing them

Most Child-to-Child and Child-to-Community activities are still small scale, but there are many of them and many success stories which need to be shared. In any country there may be a number of quite separate initiatives. For example, the Child-to-Child Trust lists eight in Kenya, seven in Indonesia, nine in Nigeria, six in Brazil and over 30 in India. Even countries with much smaller populations such as Nepal, Sudan, Zambia or Nicaragua have several separate programmes. Many countries have held national seminars so that each can benefit from others' experience.

3. One step at a time

Experience suggests that although all health priorities are important, programmes are more effective if the power and initiative of children are directed towards a limited number of health topics at one time.

- **Children can be mobilized to help on particular national campaigns:**
    - ☐ Immunization (Togo).
    - ☐ AIDS awareness (Uganda).
    - ☐ Safety (Denmark).

- **Children in projects can be directed by health workers towards action on a small number of key priorities:**
  - In a successful programme in a low-income area of Bombay, priorities chosen were anaemia, scabies and diarrhoea.
- **At school level, children and their teachers together choose a priority:**
  - In one Zambian school they chose personal hygiene and malaria.
  - In one Kenyan school: road safety and nutrition.
  - In one English school: unsafe and contaminated environment.

  In every case other priorities are taken up once one programme has been completed.

4. Co-operation and information

Communication and co-operation are keys to the success of a programme:

Between nationally and locally initiated programmes.

Between sectors especially education and health.

Between national and international agencies, and voluntary bodies such as NGOs, churches and community initiated projects.

5. Where can action be taken?

In national programmes for health education

Add in a Child-to-Child and Child-to-Community component to strengthen the programme ... as in Guinea.*

Within national curriculum policies

Agree *Facts for Life* and accept the principle of involving children as partners in spreading these.

Identify which facts children need to know at which age.

The curriculum centre then plans the integration of the facts across its curriculum within 'carrier subjects' such as science and 'support subjects' such as language and mathematics.

Suggestions for children's action are included in subject programmes ... as in Zambia.

---

*For further information about the activities in different countries mentioned on pages 33, 34 and 36, please contact the Child-to-Child Trust.

When materials are produced

Incorporate suggestions for child-involved activities within recommended teachers' and children's material for health education. Possibly highlight these activities by using the Child-to-Child logo ... as in Uganda.

Such materials for children and teachers need not be confined to health education. Story books incorporating *Facts for Life* messages have been widely produced and are read by millions of children.

At teachers' colleges

Prepare trainee or serving teachers in both facts and approaches. Colleges set up their own student-led health committees. Colleges can be linked to neighbouring schools and help to plan and monitor their child health action programmes ... as in Sierra Leone.

At school and community level

Encourage schools or groups of schools to make individual school health action plans in co-operation or consultation with health workers, as in Tanzania (Zanzibar) and other East African countries.

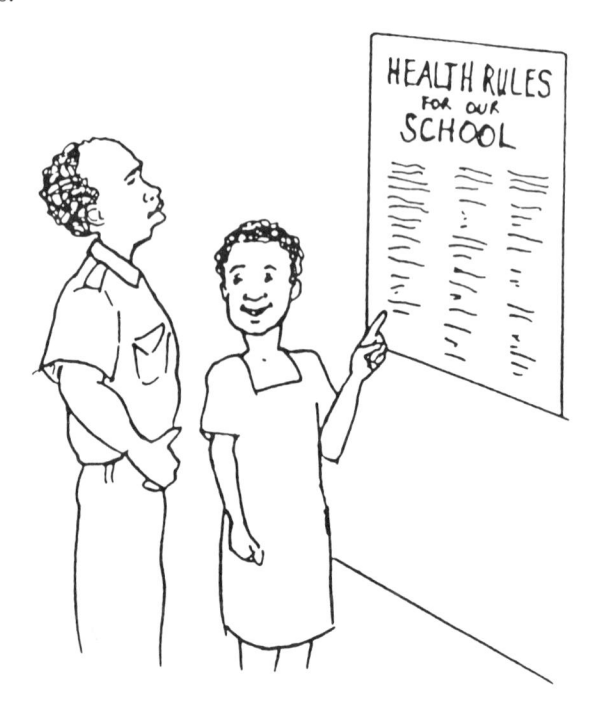

A SCHOOL HEALTH ACTION PLAN

Schools identify and plan their own implementation of *Facts for Life* priorities in consultation with their communities.

Plans can be generated by a single school, by a group of schools or by schools co-ordinated by a teachers' college.

Choosing priorities

Priorities are chosen by the head, staff and children of the school in consultation with local health workers and community leaders. Often a school aims to cover all or most of the *Facts for Life* messages but emphasizes them a few at a time.

Making a plan

The plan for a term, semester, or year includes four elements:

- Teaching vital health facts, usually through carrier subjects such as science. These may be reinforced by short, intensive 'health information spots' at regular intervals.
- Reinforcing these messages across the curriculum, e.g. in mathematics, making budgets for good nutrition, weighing children and recording their weights; in language, writing stories and plays about caring for people with AIDS.
- Action at school level, e.g. in cleanliness, nutrition, safety.
- Action planned from school to community, e.g. a campaign on immunization.

The plan in action

Once the plan is in action it is monitored by the school staff and facilitated by a health committee in which the girls and boys take a leading part.

In many schools pupils are 'twinned', with older children specifically charged with the care and instruction of younger ones.

School and community

The school-based plan is complemented by community action and community health education so that children are seen as just one vital element alongside others in changing knowledge, attitudes and practice.

Supporting the initiatives

The initiatives taken by schools do not go unrecognized. They are supported by advice, training and materials from the ministries of education and health at national level, and encouraged by local managers, advisers and inspectors.

From school

Schools can set up and encourage extra-curricular groups to act as child health workers to spread messages and take action in communities. Local school health advisers monitor and take responsibility for these groups ... as in Indonesia.

Outside school

Preschool children's groups can be helped by older children especially in child development but also to learn simple hygiene and safety through games and songs ... as in India (Gujarat state).

Local health scout programmes can involve children who have not attended or who no longer attend school ... as in Guatemala.

Children in specially difficult circumstances need also to be partners in receiving and providing *Facts for Life*: refugee children; street and working children; children in institutions; children who are disabled. Taking action to pass on these messages empowers these children ... as in Pakistan, Philippines, Romania, and Mexico.

6. Evaluation

We have suggested that involving children as partners in spreading *Facts for Life* can benefit many people. If we are to prove this we need to evaluate what changes have resulted from the actions that have been taken. In order to assess changes, we need if possible to find out and describe what existed in the first place. Thus evaluation needs to take place 'before' as well as 'after'. When this is not possible we may be able to compare outcomes, e.g. between somewhere which has undertaken a new programme and somewhere else which has not. In other cases it will be valuable to describe how an activity is being carried out and the effects which it is having. The best evaluations often contain all three kinds of evidence.

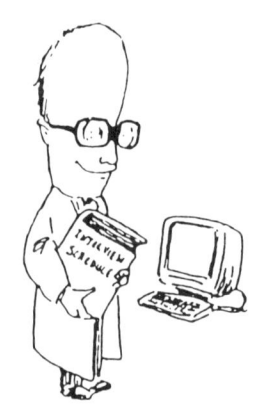

People often think of evaluation being done by people like this...

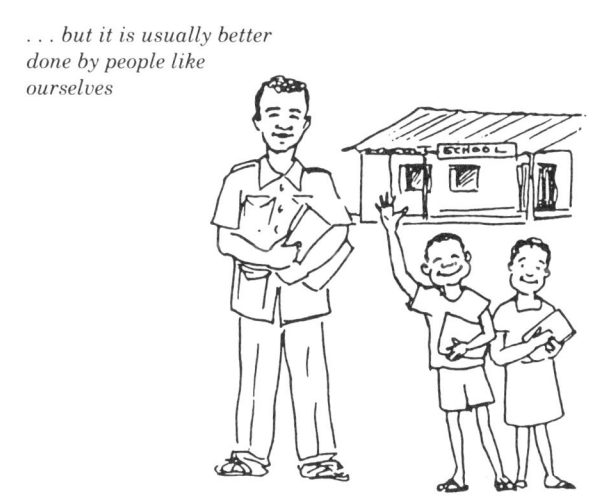

... but it is usually better done by people like ourselves

It is important to remember that evaluation is not a technical activity generally undertaken by experts. It is, rather, a way of finding out information which different kinds of people need to know. Through evaluation we can learn from our failures as well as our successes.

Measuring the effects

Finding our whether a programme is well organized and popular is relatively easy. Finding out whether a programme has made a difference is not, however, a straightforward task.

Some effects are quite easy to measure:

What facts have been learnt.

What skills have been acquired.

What actions have been taken ... immediately following the activities which have been organized.

Other effects are more difficult to measure but still possible if we do it in the right way:

Whether knowledge and skills are *retained* over a period of time. This can be measured by retesting.

Whether attitudes have changed – this is best measured through indicators such as interest (attends health club) or actions (always washes hands).

The most difficult effect to measure is whether the activities have resulted in changes in the health status of those who undertook them and those who received the messages.

It is extremely hard to say whether children's activities were responsible for the effect, or partly responsible, or whether the effect was caused by something else entirely. It is much better to be honest but cautious in our claims, e.g.:

Children in five schools in the community concentrated on a clean water campaign in which they also spread messages on oral rehydration. During the year there was a radio and poster campaign. The health centre reported a 30 per cent drop in cases of young children with serious dehydration and only seven deaths as against 11 in the same season in the previous year.

The schools concluded that their campaign had probably made some difference.

How do we evaluate?

Most methods of evaluation can be used by anyone who organizes a programme or uses an activity. Indeed they are actions we do every day. We evaluate by:

- **Asking questions** (often comparing answers to questions asked *before* an activity with answers to the same questions asked *after* it):

    Written questions:
    ▫ Are children's stools more or less likely to spread disease than adult ones?

    Oral questions:
    ▫ How can you recognize the danger signs of pneumonia?

- **Observing and recording:**
    ▫ Are more water pots covered?
    ▫ Do children play with babies more? Have they made any toys?

- **Practical tests:**
    ▫ Asking people to use and read a growth monitoring scale and chart.

- **Meetings and discussion:**
    ▫ Letting people talk freely about what they have observed or done gives much information, e.g. discussions at a parent/teacher meeting about what children have said and done.

- **Using written material:**
    ▫ Keeping and consulting diaries and records, e.g. minutes of school health committee; records of health club.

- **Games and role-playing:**
    ▫ Setting a problem and noting responses, e.g. A person with AIDS is shunned by other people in the neighbourhood. What would you do if this happened?

What do we evaluate?

We need to evaluate the effects of activities on the *children who carry them out*.

For example:

- **Changes in knowledge**

  Before starting the unit on coughs, colds and pneumonia, all the children were tested. Seventy per cent thought that colds could be treated by medicines from the market and only 10 per cent mentioned the danger signs of pneumonia.

  Later two classes were tested (six weeks after they had been given the information). In both, the belief in market medicines had decreased but the results of the question on signs of pneumonia were very interesting. In one class where the teacher had given the information on the blackboard only 45 per cent of children had remembered it correctly. In another the children had made pendulums with a stone and string (see page 130) to count fast breathing; 90 per cent of children remembered the message.

- **Changes in skills**

  As a result of the first aid activities in the Red Cross club, children gained a number of practical skills and gained badges once they passed their aptitude tests.

  However, the club organizer was also interested to discover whether they had gained skills in observation and problem solving. It seemed from a survey of parents that some children were noticing hazards at home and taking action, particularly in the kitchen. ('Can we put up a shelf to keep those bottles out of baby's reach?')

- **Changes in attitudes and behaviour**

  *Health workers, youth leaders and project organizers had a long discussion on how to evaluate attitudes. They all agreed that tests were not likely to be useful for this. Finally they made a list of some of the ways of behaving (*indicators*) which they should look for in children, e.g.:*

  ☐ *Attends health club regularly.*

  ☐ *Notices and reports poor hygiene or safety hazards.*

  ☐ *Makes a toy for baby, etc.*

  Making the list taught them a lot about what to look for and encourage.

Note: A guide to evaluation entitled *Doing it Better*, published by the Child-to-Child Trust, helps those who work with children to understand simple evaluation techniques. Available from TALC, address on page 183.

We also need to evaluate the effects of children's activities on *their families, schools and communities.*
For example:

- **Changes in knowledge**

    Children, helped by their teachers and club organizers, were invited to design their own knowledge tests both for other children and for some adults at home (where they agreed to take part). They made simple questions, pictures, and a story about diarrhoea with gaps in it for people to fill in either orally or in writing. They found this difficult but learnt a great deal by doing it. They were helped by project organizers.

    In some cases, these questions were the same as those which they had asked right at the beginning of the project. From asking these questions they discovered that most children and some parents had gained a good deal of knowledge, but additional questions showed that some of the messages had not been properly understood. (Some people thought that the oral rehydration drink was a 'medicine' to be taken in small quantities.)

- **Changes in practice**

    After the health scouts had visited families in the community regularly (each pair was responsible for five families), the health worker herself visited a sample of families and talked to mothers. She found that many more of them were cooking green vegetables daily with their main meal.

- **Changes in health status**

    After the school had finished the activity, the health worker waited for three months and then compared her records with those of the same period last year. 'I can't say for certain that it is the result of your Child-to-Child project on safety,' she told the children, 'but what I can say is that fewer babies have been brought into the health centre with burns than during the same time last year.'

- **Changes in approaches at school**

    In the project schools, children were 'paired' with older children responsible for the hygiene and safety of the younger ones. Older children also had responsibilities in the health committees.

    A survey made over a number of schools reported a considerable improvement in hygiene ... both older and younger children had gained skills (e.g. older children had taught younger ones how to clean their teeth more thoroughly and, in so doing, learnt a lot themselves).

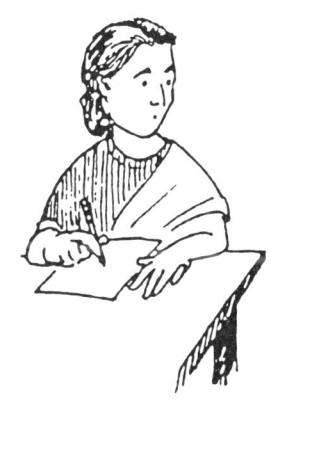

My school brother never checked my fingernails today

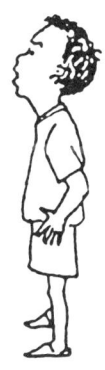

Some comments also reflected that older children were getting more skilful in helping the younger ones help themselves (instead of just telling them what to do).

- **Changes in participation**

A group from the curriculum centre was appointed to visit a number of schools, colleges and health scout programmes in different areas. In one district, far more activity was noted than another. Questioning revealed that:

☐ *The organizing committee was more active.*

☐ *A local in-service centre was particularly involved and interested.*

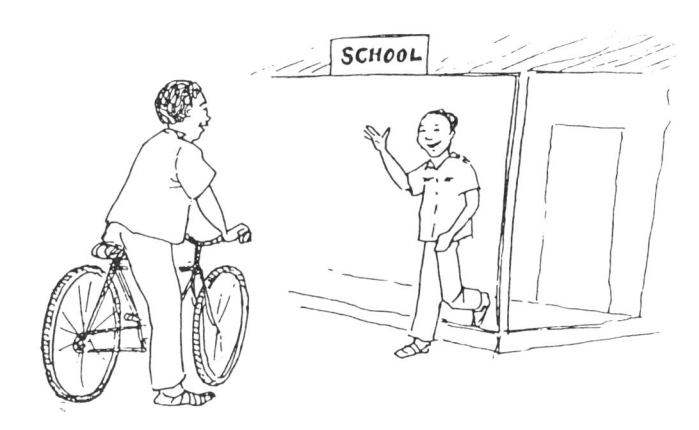

☐ *Transport was available to visit schools and clubs.*

Visits were arranged so that others could come to the area to see the good work that was going on.

Are the approaches well planned and managed?

At the same time as looking at the outcomes of new approaches, we need to ask whether they are well *planned* and well *managed*. Experience with many programmes suggests that the following questions need to be asked at the planning stage:

Do those who seek to implement the approach really understand it? Are they committed to it? Do they respect children?

Is what we are expecting of children reasonable, feasible and interesting for children to do?

Do the new approaches complement and fit into other health programmes and priorities?

Has necessary co-ordination and co-operation been foreseen and planned between health and education sectors?

When the programme is *implemented* we may need to ask the following:

Are the original goals being kept in mind? Are children remaining in the centre of the activity and continuing to be given responsibility?

Is management efficient and cost-effective?

Are approaches being well adapted to local needs and cultures?

Is the right training being provided to the right people?

Are those who undertake the programme (including the children) monitoring activities and changing their programme as a result?

Who finds the answers to these questions?

These questions all need to be asked and answered by those who plan and organize programmes, but there will be occasions when they will need to ask *outsiders* for help. These outsiders do not always have to be specialists in evaluation.

They can be:

Doctors and other health workers, who can check whether the messages are correct and whether health has improved.

Administrators and planners, who can assess whether activities are cost-effective.

Community leaders and community members, who can be asked to judge whether attitudes or actions of children or the community have changed.

Remember: Experts are often needed to help us find the answers to some of the questions we ask, but many different people are experts in different things. Often children themselves are the best experts we can find.

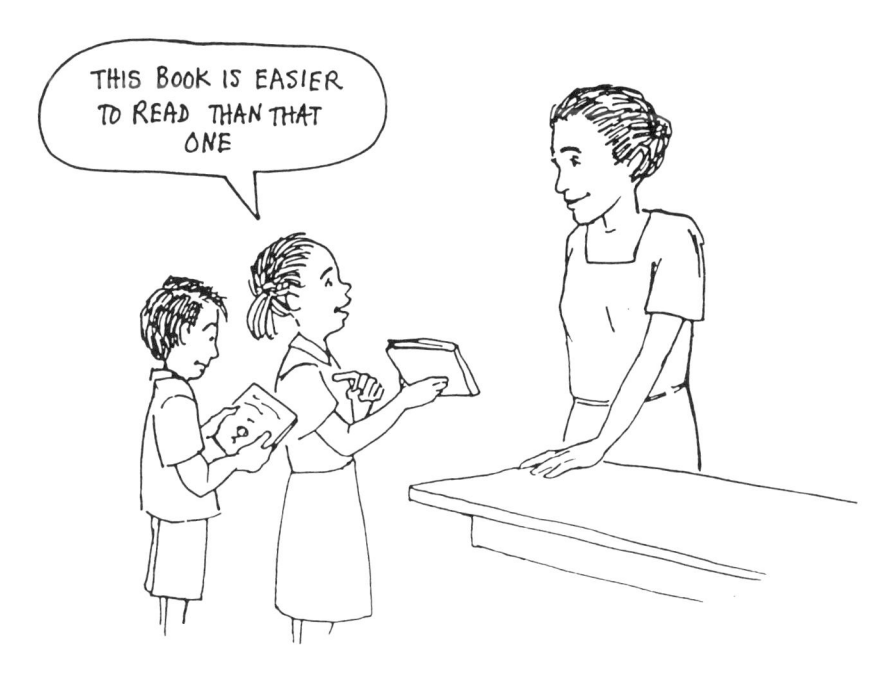

THIS BOOK IS EASIER TO READ THAN THAT ONE

Children for health?

Are there some things we do not need to measure? Evaluating and measuring is necessary but takes time. Certain effects must be measured, but do we have to prove that children co-operate better in families if they help to improve the health of their brothers and sisters?

Do we have to prove that schools serve their communities better if they teach their children to meet health problems in their communities?

Do we need to prove that someone learns a fact or skill better if he has to teach it to someone else?

Do we need to be persuaded that child citizens whose concern is directed towards improvement of their neighbourhood become better citizens?

We do not! These are truths we all know from experience.

Our problem, therefore, is not *whether* child action for *Facts for Life* is valuable. It is rather that we need to examine *how* children can best be served and how they can best serve their communities.

PART TWO

Health Messages and Children's Action

**Breastfeeding
Child Growth
Child Development
Hygiene
Diarrhoea
Immunization
Coughs and Colds
Malaria
AIDS
Safe Motherhood
Accidents*
Food for the Family***

*These sections have been specially prepared for *Children for Health*.

TWELVE MESSAGES TO SAVE AND IMPROVE LIFE

In this part we show what health ideas children need to know and pass on about the prime messages from *Facts for Life*. We have added two messages which are essential for children to know and around which many activities can be developed. The prime messages appear as they are in *Facts for Life* but in a few cases the supporting information has been shortened. The text of Timing Births has been incorporated into Safe Motherhood. The text of Malaria has been expanded to include more information on Nursing Children with Fever.

Each of the 12 sections has:

- **The prime message and supporting information**

The supporting information provides a great deal of background knowledge for teachers and health workers.

- **Objectives**

These summarize what children should know and be able to do.

- **Activities for understanding**

There are many activities that teachers can do with children to help them understand important health ideas. We have selected a small number of activities that work well and which are examples of different methods that help children learn. E.g. Dehydration is an important idea which is made easier to understand if children do an experiment that shows how babies lose fluids when they have diarrhoea.

- **Activities for taking action**

As well as understanding health messages, it is important for children to be able to apply and pass on what they have learnt. We have chosen activities that show what children can do, by themselves or together, to contribute to their own health and that of others in their families, schools and neighbourhood.

- **A range of methods**

Activities have been chosen because they represent a range of methods which can be used. It is very likely that those described in full in one section may be also useful in another, even though they do not appear there, e.g. techniques for interviews, story-writing, surveys, and using pictures to promote discussion may be useful in almost every section.

- **A 'basket of ideas'**
In each section there is a 'basket of ideas' which can be developed by those working with children. You will be able to think of many more activities that both promote understanding and help children to take action for health.

- **Evaluation questions**
At the end of each section there are evaluation questions to help children, teachers and health workers ask themselves how well they remember and use what they have learnt, and whether their actions were effective.

Messages reinforce each other
Many messages in *Facts for Life* overlap because different aspects of health influence each other. *It is therefore important, when preparing activities on one theme, e.g. Diarrhoea, to read through and study both the information and the activities in related themes, e.g. Hygiene and Breastfeeding.*

What children need to know and pass on about
Breastfeeding

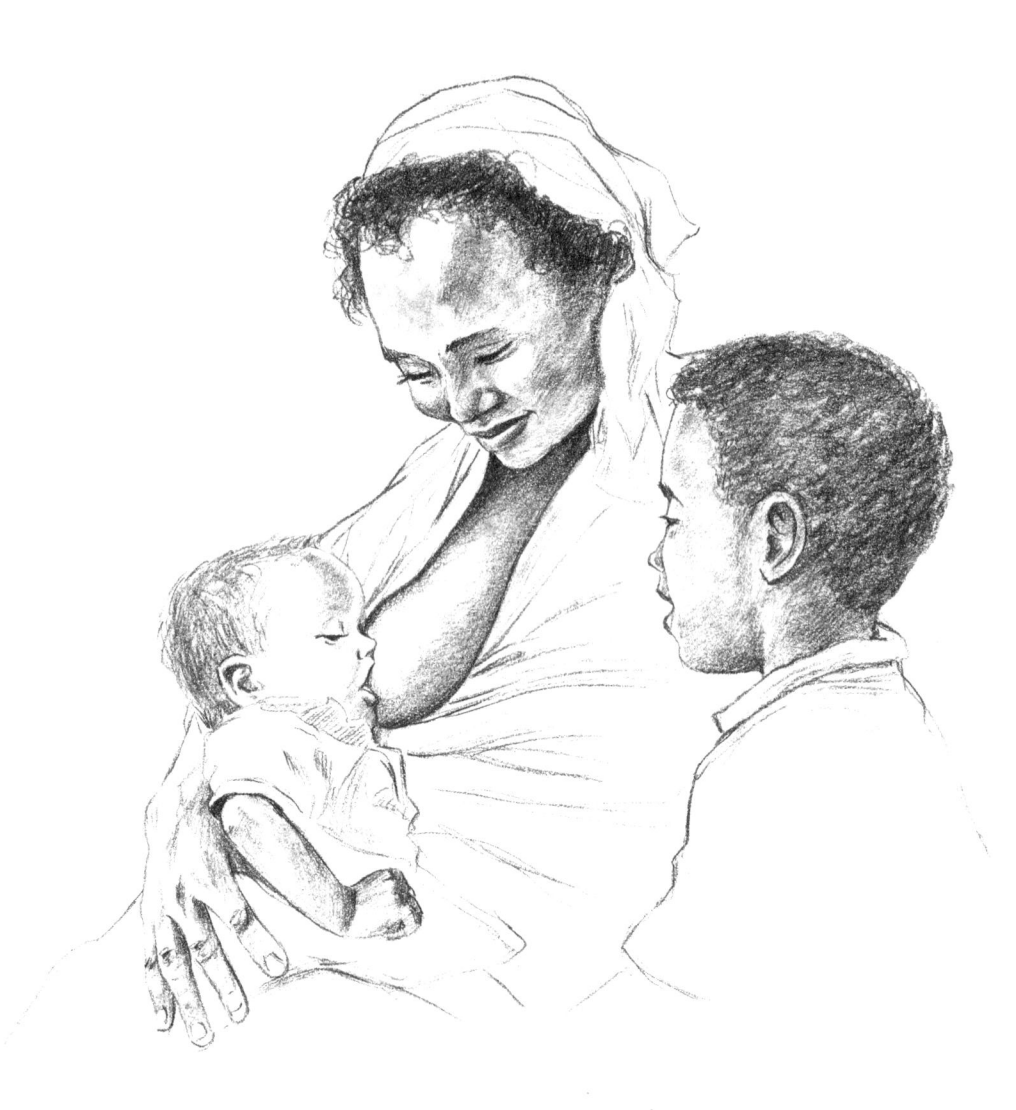

Babies fed on breastmilk have fewer illnesses and less malnutrition than babies who are bottle-fed on other foods. If all babies were exclusively breastfed for about the first six months of life, then the deaths of more than one million infants a year would be prevented.

Bottle-feeding is a special threat in poor communities where parents may not be able to afford sufficient milk-powder, may not have clean water to mix it with, and may not be able to sterilize teats and feeding bottles.

The six prime messages in this chapter can help to avert that threat and promote the healthy growth of young children. Children need to be aware of these messages because they are the next generation of mothers and fathers. They can also help spread these messages in the communities in which they live as well as being especially helpful to their mothers at home when they are breastfeeding babies.

Activities in this section should be related to those in Child Growth and Food for the Family.

PRIME MESSAGES
and supporting information

1 Breastmilk alone is the best possible food and drink for a baby. No other food or drink is needed for about the first six months of life.

● From the moment of birth up to the age of about six months, breastmilk is all the food and drink a baby needs. It is the best food a child will ever have. All substitutes, including cow's milk, infant formula, milk-powder solutions, and cereal gruels, are inferior.

● Even in hot, dry climates, breastmilk contains sufficient water for a young baby's needs. Additional water or sugary drinks are not needed to quench the baby's thirst. They can also be harmful. If the baby is also given water, or drinks made with water, then the risk of getting diarrhoea and other illnesses increases.

● Other foods and drinks are necessary when a baby reaches the age of about six months. If monthly weighing shows that a child under six months of age is not growing well, then the child may need more frequent breastfeeding. If the child is already being breastfed frequently, then lack of weight gain shows either that the child has an illness or that other foods, in addition to breastmilk, are now necessary.

● Until the age of nine or ten months, the baby should be breastfed before other foods are given. Breastfeeding should continue well into the second year of life – and for longer if possible.

2 | **Babies should start to breastfeed as soon as possible after birth. Virtually every mother can breastfeed her baby.**

● Mothers and newborn babies should not be put in different rooms. The baby should be allowed to suck at the breast as often as he or she wants.

● If a mother gives birth in a maternity unit, then she has a right to expect that her newborn baby will be kept near her in the same room, 24 hours a day, and that no other food or drink will be given to her baby except breastmilk.

● Starting to breastfeed immediately after birth stimulates the production of breastmilk. Breastfeeding should begin not later than one hour after the delivery of the baby.

● The thick yellowish milk (called colostrum) that the mother produces in the first few days after birth is good for babies. It is nutritious and helps to protect them against common infections. The baby does not need any other food or drink while waiting for the mother's milk to 'come in'. In some countries, mothers are advised not to feed this colostrum to their babies. This advice is wrong.

● Many mothers need help when they begin to breastfeed, especially if the baby is their first. An experienced and sympathetic adviser, such as a woman who has successfully breastfed, can help a mother avoid or solve many common problems.

● Almost all mothers can produce enough milk if:

  □ The baby takes the breast into his or her mouth in a good position.

  □ The baby sucks as often, and for as long, as he or she wants, including during the night.

● Crying is not a sign that a baby needs artificial feeds. It normally means that the baby needs to be held and cuddled more. Some babies need to suck the breast simply for comfort. If the baby is hungry, more sucking will produce more breastmilk.

● Mothers who are not confident that they have enough breastmilk often give their babies other food or drink in the first few months of life. But this means that the baby sucks at the breast less often. So less breastmilk is produced. To stop this happening, mothers need to be reassured that they can feed their young babies properly with *breastmilk alone*. They need the encouragement and practical support of their families, the child's father, neighbours, friends, health workers and women's organizations.

● Husbands, families, and communities can help to protect the health of both mothers and babies by making sure that the mother has enough food and by helping with her many tiring tasks.

● Breastfeeding can be an opportunity for a mother to take a few minutes of much-needed rest. Husbands or other family members can help by encouraging the mother to lie down, in peace and quiet, while she breastfeeds her baby.

3 | **Breastfeeding causes more milk to be produced. A baby needs to suck frequently at the breast so that enough breastmilk is produced to meet the baby's needs.**

● From birth, the baby should breastfeed whenever he or she wants to – often indicated by crying. Frequent sucking at the breast is necessary to stimulate the production of more breastmilk.

● 'Topping up' breastmilk feeds with milk-powder solutions, infant formulas, cow's milk, water, or other drinks, reduces the amount of milk the baby takes from the breast. This leads to less breastmilk being produced. The use of a bottle to give other drinks can cause the baby to stop breastfeeding completely. It can also confuse the baby because the sucking action of bottle-feeding is very different from sucking at the breast. Babies who are confused between sucking at the breast and sucking at the bottle may drink less breastmilk. This will cause less breastmilk to be produced.

4 | **Breastfeeding helps to protect babies and young children against dangerous diseases. Bottle-feeding can lead to serious illness and death.**

● Breastmilk is the baby's first 'immunization'. It helps to protect the baby against diarrhoea, coughs and colds, and other common illnesses. The protection is greatest when breastmilk alone is given to the baby for about the first six months.

● Cow's milk, infant formulas, milk-powder solutions, maize gruel and other infant foods do not give babies any special protection against diarrhoea, coughs and colds, and other diseases.

● Bottle-feeding can cause illnesses such as diarrhoea unless the water is boiled and the bottle and teats are sterilized in boiling water before each feed. The more often a child is ill, the more likely it is that he or she will become malnourished. That is why, in a community without clean drinking water, a bottle-fed baby is many times more likely to die of diarrhoea than a baby fed exclusively on breastmilk for about the first six months.

● Mothers should be helped to breastfeed their babies. If for any reason a mother does not breastfeed, then she should be helped in other ways to give her baby good nutrition and protection against disease.

● The best food for a baby who, for whatever reason, cannot be breastfed, is milk squeezed from the mother's breast. It should be given in a cup that has been very well cleaned. Cups are safer than bottles and teats because they are easier to keep clean.

● The best food for any baby whose own mother's milk is not available is the breastmilk of another mother.

● If non-human milk has to be used, it should be given from a clean cup rather than a bottle. Milk-powder solutions should be prepared using water that has been boiled and then cooled.

● Cow's milk, infant formula, or milk-powder solutions can cause poor growth if too much water is added in order to make it go further.

● Cow's milk and milk-powder solutions go bad if left to stand at room temperature for a few hours. Breastmilk can be stored for at least eight hours at room temperature without going bad.

● In low-income communities, the cost of cow's milk or powdered milk, plus bottles, teats, and the fuel for boiling water, can be as much as 25-50% of a family's income.

5 | **A variety of additional foods is necessary when a child is about six months old, but breastfeeding should continue well into the second year of a child's life and for longer if possible.**

● Although children need additional foods after about the first six months of life, breastmilk is still an important source of energy and protein, and other nutrients such as vitamin A, and helps to protect against disease during the child's second year of life.

● Babies get ill frequently as they learn to crawl, walk, and play. A child who is ill needs breastmilk. It provides a nutritious, easily digestible food when the child loses appetite for other foods.

● Between the ages of one and two, a baby benefits from breastmilk as well as needing family foods. Breastfeeding is good for the child as part of a meal, or between meals, or whenever the child feels hungry. But at this time, all children need other foods. In the second year of life, breastfeeding should be an addition to, not a substitute for, normal meals.

● Breastfeeding also comforts a child when he or she is frightened, hurt, angry, or tearful.

6 | **Breastfeeding gives a mother 98% protection against pregnancy for six months after giving birth – *if* her baby breastfeeds frequently, day and night, *if* the baby is not regularly given other food and drink, and *if* the mother's periods have not returned.**

N.B. Some of the supporting information included in *Facts for Life* has been omitted or shortened.

OBJECTIVES for children's understanding and action

Children should:

● Understand the benefits of breastfeeding. Breastmilk provides all the food and drink a baby needs for about the first six months of life, and protects against disease.

● Understand the dangers of bottle-feeding and how it can lead to disease and malnutrition.

● Understand the importance of slowly introducing foods at about six months while carrying on breastfeeding until beyond the second birthday.

● Know how to prepare food for babies from about six months.

● Know how to help breastfeeding mothers by taking care of younger children.

UNDERSTANDING about breastfeeding and first food for babies

1. An interview and discussion ... How long did you feed me? What was my first food?

Make a list of questions

Ask children what questions they will ask their mothers to find out how they were fed as babies. Write some of the questions on the blackboard. Children decide which questions relate to very young babies and which questions relate to older babies. Then they put the questions in a sequence. The final list might look like this:

- How long was I breastfed?
- When did I first start having food as well as breastmilk?
- What kind of food did you give me for my first food? Is it the same for boys and girls?
- How old was I when I began eating full family meals?
- How often in the day did I have food as well as breastmilk?
- How old was I when I stopped having breastmilk?

Plan the interview

Children write out the list of questions they will ask. Remind them to save some space to record the answers. Help them to decide:

- What is the best time for mother to answer my questions?
- What will I say to mother to explain why I want to know about this?

Use the information from the interviews

Ask children to tell the class about the results of their interviews. Help them to compare their findings. Follow this with a discussion. Ask children to record and learn the main health messages about feeding babies.

2. Learning by reading graphs ... comparing deaths of children who are breastfed and bottle-fed

Draw a graph on the blackboard or a piece of paper and then ask questions about the information on it to help children think about the reasons why bottle-feeding is so dangerous.

Sample questions on the graph:

- How many bottle-fed babies died?
- How many breastfed babies died?

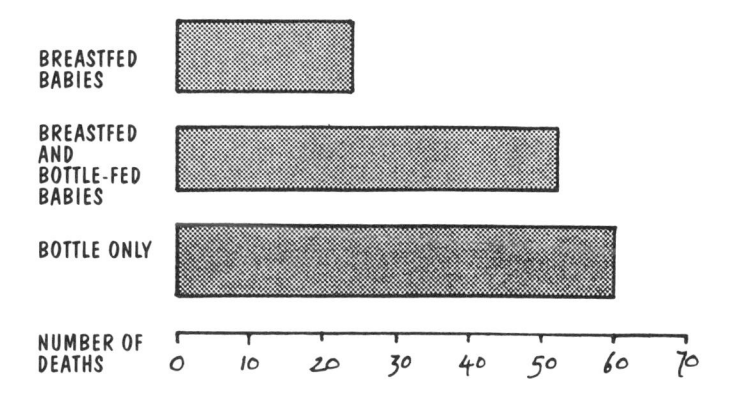

Bar chart showing number of deaths by feeding type:
- BREASTFED BABIES: ~20
- BREASTFED AND BOTTLE-FED BABIES: ~50
- BOTTLE ONLY: ~65

NUMBER OF DEATHS axis: 0, 10, 20, 30, 40, 50, 60, 70

- How many more bottle-fed babies died than breastfed babies?
- Why do you think there is this difference?
- How would you like your baby to be fed?

3. Learning from stories ... breastfed babies are healthier

- Make up stories, or adapt stories using characters well known in the culture: stories could contrast the experience of two mothers, one who breastfed her baby and one who (for one reason or another) decided to bottle-feed. Remember to present these reasons sympathetically – mothers who bottle-feed nearly always do so because they believe it is the best way to help their families.

- Use incomplete stories and let children complete them. Here are two:

  A mother who is quite poor went to town and had her baby there. She stayed with friends for three weeks afterwards. Soon after the baby was born someone gave her some milk-powder and persuaded her to start feeding her baby with a bottle. After three weeks she went back to the village ...

  ... When the baby was four months old it was very thin and suffered from diarrhoea.

  What happened in between?

  A mother in town got a full-time job when her baby was two months old. She decided to employ a childminder who had not been to school. She gave her a bottle and showed her how to clean it and feed the baby with it.

  What happened later?

- Discuss the stories based on children's experience. If many children have been involved in making up stories or completing stories, collect different versions and compare them.

    In particular, discuss:
    - Why do breastfed babies grow up healthier?
    - Why do mothers bottle-feed instead of breastfeed? (e.g. Because they received poor advice, or insufficient support.)
    - What are the dangers of bottle-feeding?
    - If mothers do not breastfeed, what are some of the ways in which babies can be kept healthier? (*Use supporting information on page 52 as a reference.*)

4. An enquiry and discussion ... how much does it cost to bottle-feed a baby?

Find out from the health worker what milk-powders are most commonly used locally to make up feeding bottles for babies.

Get a tin of milk-powder and discuss with children the instructions for making up the feed. Help children to calculate:

- How long a tin lasts when a baby is fed according to the instructions.
- How much it costs to feed a baby on milk-powder for a week, and compare this to what families earn.

Are there other costs (e.g. for bottles, teats, firewood)? Discuss what can happen if families cannot afford all this money.

5. Looking carefully at advertisements ... what do they want us to think (and buy)?

In most countries advertisements for milk-powder for babies are no longer permitted on radio or television, or in public places.

However, there are many advertisements for prepared supplementary foods for babies. While these foods may be nutritious, they are expensive and no improvement on home-prepared foods.

Advertisements may also suggest that mothers introduce these foods far too early.

Children observe, describe and discuss advertisements appearing in public places or on food labels. Here is an example:

WHAT IS THIS ADVERTISEMENT TRYING TO MAKE US THINK?

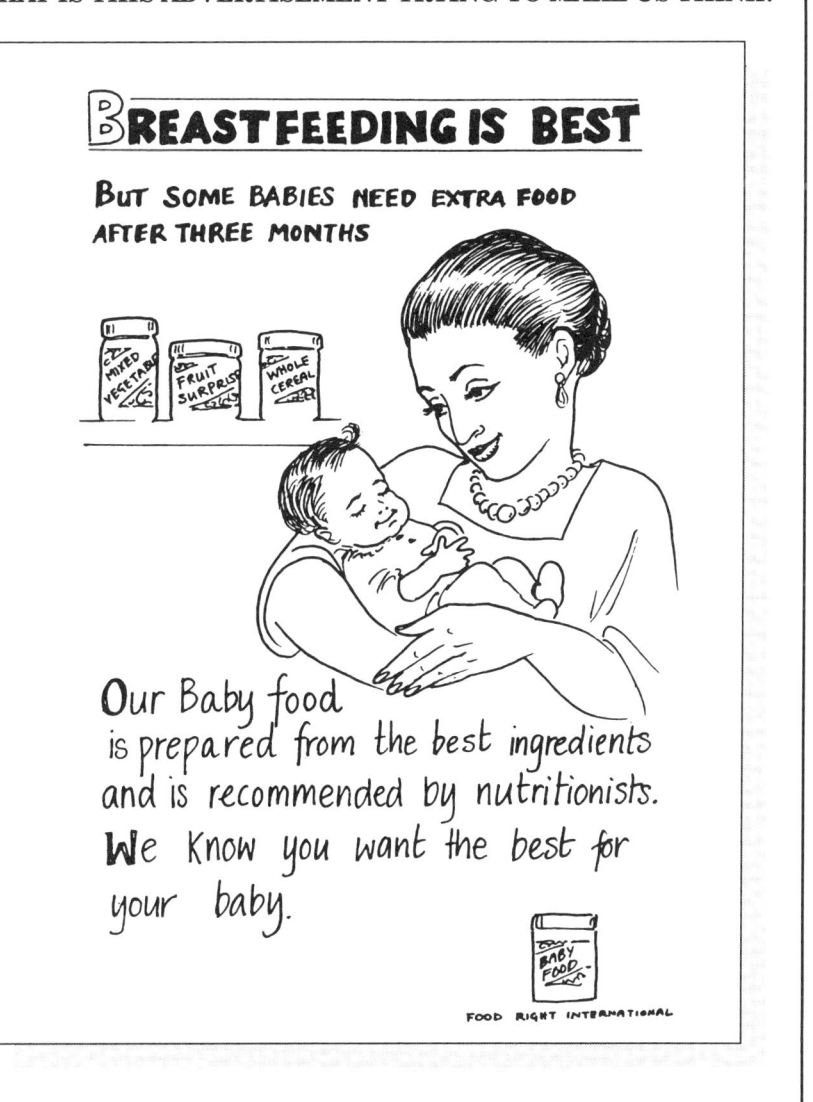

> # BREASTFEEDING IS BEST
>
> BUT SOME BABIES NEED EXTRA FOOD AFTER THREE MONTHS
>
> [MIXED VEGETABLES] [FRUIT SURPRISE] [WHOLE CEREAL]
>
> Our Baby food is prepared from the best ingredients and is recommended by nutritionists. We know you want the best for your baby.
>
> [BABY FOOD]
>
> FOOD RIGHT INTERNATIONAL

Ask children to describe what the advertisement contains, and analyze how it tries to persuade mothers to buy the product. Look at both the pictures and the wording, e.g. a successful, well-dressed mother; words such as 'recommended by nutritionists'.

Is the wording trying to make mothers feel they may not be feeding their babies properly? e.g. 'Extra food after three months'; 'the best for your baby'.

6. Demonstration and discussion ... preparing food for young babies

Children prepare and cook some food suitable for a baby of about six months, using the ingredients below or other high-energy mixtures that are given to young babies locally. This recipe is from Africa and is also suitable for older babies.

Banana and potato purée

Ingredients

Cooking banana	1 large
Oil or margarine	1 teaspoon
Potato	1 large
Green leafy vegetables	half cup chopped (i.e. 3 small leaves of kale)

Method

Wash, peel and cut up the banana and potato.
Wash and cut up the vegetables.
Boil everything together in one cup of water in a covered pan for 15 minutes or until well cooked.
Mash and pass through a sieve.
Serve warm.

This makes about one cup of cooked food. A young baby will only eat a few spoonfuls of this at one mealtime, after breastfeeding.

After the activity of making the food, children can:
- Describe the taste.
- Describe why the vegetables are washed and peeled and why the food is mashed.
- Write a description of the steps they followed. Make it at home for the baby.
- Report on whether the baby liked it or not.

CHILDREN'S ACTION
I Can

● Help mother when she is breastfeeding the baby by amusing other children.

● Help mother by doing jobs to let her have time to rest.

● Know how to prepare different kinds of baby foods and help feed the baby when he or she starts other food in addition to breastmilk.

We Can

● Put on a play that tells how a baby got diarrhoea from bottle-feeding; present it to the neighbours.

- Make a class book of recipes for baby foods and display it, and the foods, at a school open day.
- Make and display a poster: *'Dangers of bottle-feeding'*.

BASKET OF IDEAS

- The health worker or nursing sister explains to older children what can happen when small babies do not have enough of the right mixture of foods.
- Children grow special foods for babies (e.g. vegetables or fruit).
- Children demonstrate how to keep a baby's cup and spoon clean.

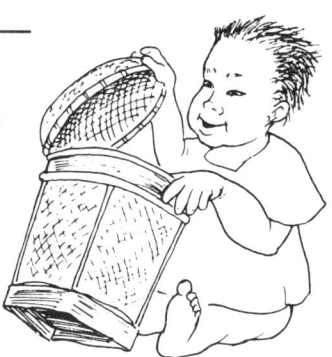

EVALUATION QUESTIONS

Children
- What have I done to help my mother or aunt who is breastfeeding a baby?

Teachers
- Can children list the advantages of breastfeeding and the dangers of bottle-feeding?
- Do children know how to prepare high-energy food for babies?

Health Workers
- Did we use children's posters in our 'breast is best' campaign?

What children need to know and pass on about
Child Growth

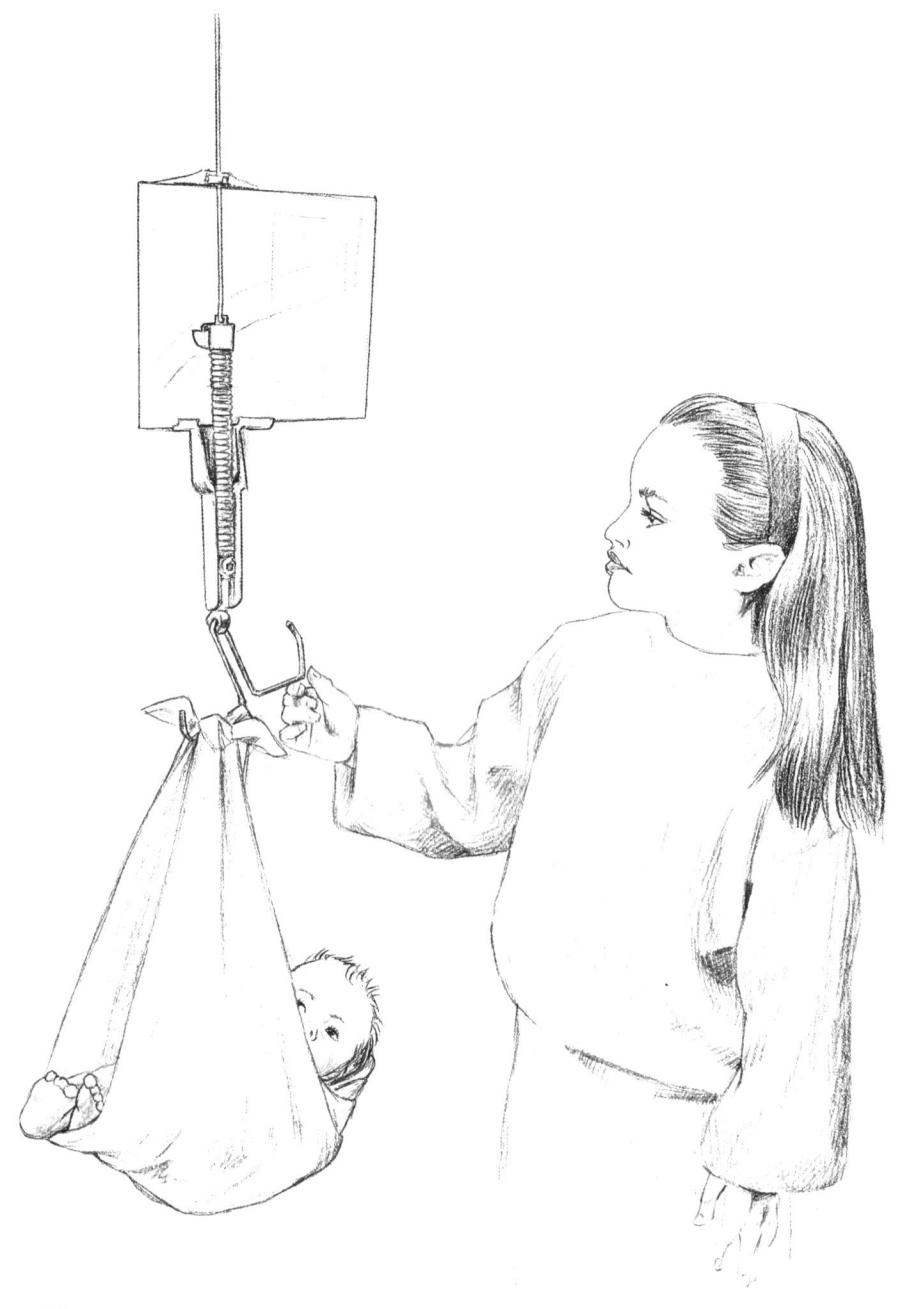

Malnutrition and infection hold back the physical growth of millions of children. If children are not properly fed when they are small, their mental growth also suffers.

Sometimes parents are unable to feed their children properly because of drought, famine, war or poverty.

But sometimes it is possible to improve child growth by better knowledge and better practice. Older children often care for their younger brothers and sisters; sometimes they have gained knowledge in school which their families lack. They can therefore help greatly in promoting more frequent feeding of small children, in weighing and measuring them, and in recognizing danger signs when they are not growing properly.

PRIME MESSAGES
and supporting information

1 Children from birth to the age of three years should be weighed every month. If there is no weight gain for two months, something is wrong.

● Regular monthly weight gain is the most important sign of a child's overall health and development. It is the child's own weight gain which is important, not how the child compares in weight to other children.

● It is therefore important to weigh young children every month. If a child does not gain weight over a two-month period, then parents and health workers should act. The child is being held back either by illness, or poor food, or lack of attention. The following paragraphs cover the most likely causes of poor growth and the most important actions parents can take to keep a child growing well.

● Breastfeeding helps protect a baby from common illnesses and ensure growth for the first few months of life. A full course of immunizations in the first year of life is also essential – it protects against diseases which cause undernutrition.

● When additional foods are given, the risk of infection increases. From now on, it is specially important to check that the child is putting on weight regularly from one month to the next. If a child under the age of three is not gaining weight, and if the child has good food, these are the 10 most important questions to ask:

- Is the child eating frequently enough? (a child should eat five or six times a day)
- Do the child's meals have too little energy in them? (small amounts of oil or fats should be added)
- Is the child frequently ill? (needs medical attention)
- Has the child been refusing to eat when ill? (needs tempting to eat when ill and extra meals to catch up afterwards)
- Is the child getting enough vitamin A? (needs dark green vegetables every day)
- Is the child being bottle-fed? (bottle and water may not be clean, sugary drinks may be being used instead of milk)
- Are food and water being kept clean? (if not, child will often be ill)
- Are faeces being put into a latrine or buried? (if not, child will often be ill)
- Does the child have worms? (needs deworming medicine from health centre)
- Is the child alone too much? (needs more stimulation and attention)

Recording the child's weight with a dot on the child's 'growth chart' and joining up the dots after each monthly weighing gives a line which enables a mother to see her child's growth. An upward line means the child is doing well. A flat line is a cause for concern. A downward line is a sure sign that all is not well with the child. A child who is given only breastmilk will almost always grow well in the first few months of life. Seeing this good progress on a growth chart helps give the mother confidence.

2 Breastmilk alone is the best possible food for about the first six months of a child's life.

● From the moment of birth up to the age of about six months, breastmilk is all the food and drink a baby needs to grow well. In these early months, when a baby is most at risk, breastmilk helps to protect against diarrhoea and other common infections.

● Breastmilk is the best food a child will ever have. If possible, breastfeeding should continue well into the second year of life and for longer if possible.

3 | **By the age of about six months, the child needs other foods in addition to breastmilk.**

● At the age of about six months, most infants need other foods in addition to breastmilk. Before the age of six months, an infant who is not gaining enough weight may need more frequent breastfeeding.
 If the child is already being breastfed frequently, then failure to gain weight shows that other foods in addition to breastmilk are now necessary.
 For an infant who continues to grow well, additional food may not be necessary until seven or even eight months. After that, all children need other foods in addition to breastmilk.

● The baby should be breastfed *before* being given other foods so that the mother will have more breastmilk for a longer period.

● Boiled, peeled and mashed vegetables should be added to a young child's gruel or other weaning food at least once each day.

● The greater the variety of foods the child eats, the better.

4 | **A child under three years of age needs food five or six times a day.**

● A child's stomach is smaller than an adult's, so a child cannot eat as much as an adult at one meal. But its energy needs, for its size, are greater. So the problem is how to get enough 'energy food' into the child. The answer is:

  ☐ Feed the child frequently – five or six times a day.
  ☐ Enrich the child's gruel or porridge with mashed vegetables and a little oil or fat.

● A child's food should not be left standing for hours. Germs can grow in it which may make the child ill. As it is usually not possible to cook fresh food for a child five or six times a day, dried foods or snacks should be given in between meals – fruits, bread, patties, biscuits, nuts, coconut, bananas or whatever clean food is easily available. Breastmilk is also an ideal 'snack' and is always clean and free from germs.

5 | **A child under three years of age needs a small amount of extra fat or oil added to the family's ordinary food.**

● The family's normal food needs to be enriched to meet the special energy needs of the child. This means adding mashed vegetables and small amounts of fats or oils – butter, ghee, vegetable oil, soya oil, coconut oil, corn oil, groundnut oil, or crushed nuts.

● Breastmilk also enriches a child's diet, and breastfeeding should continue, if possible, until well into the second year of a child's life.

6 | **All children need foods rich in vitamin A – breastmilk, green leafy vegetables, and orange-coloured fruits and vegetables.**

● Over 200,000 children go blind each year because they do not have enough vitamin A in their bodies. Vitamin A may also protect children against other illnesses such as diarrhoea. It should therefore be a part of every child's daily diet.

● Vitamin A comes from breastmilk, dark green leafy vegetables, and from orange or yellow fruits and vegetables such as carrots, papayas, and mangoes.

● If a child has had diarrhoea or measles, vitamin A will be lost from the child's body. It can be replaced by breastfeeding more often, and by feeding the child more fruit and vegetables.

7 | **After an illness, a child needs one extra meal every day for at least a week.**

● One of the most important skills of a parent is the skill of stopping illnesses from holding back a child's growth. In times of illness, and especially if the illness is diarrhoea or measles, the appetite falls and less of the food that is eaten is absorbed into the body. If this happens several times a year, the child's growth will be held back.

● So it is essential to encourage a child who is ill to eat and drink. This can be difficult if the child does not want to eat, so it is important to keep offering food the child likes, usually soft, sweet foods, a little at a time and as often as possible. Breastfeeding is especially important.

● When the illness is over, extra meals should be given so that the child catches up on the growth lost. A good rule is to give a child an extra meal every day for at least a week after the illness is over. The child is not fully recovered from an illness until he or she is at least the same weight as when the illness began.

● If illness and poor appetite persist for more than a few days, the child should be taken to a health worker.

● It is also important to protect a child's growth by preventing illness:

☐ Give a child breastmilk alone for about the first six months of life. Then introduce other foods, and continue to breastfeed.

☐ Make sure your child is fully immunized before the age of one year.

☐ Always use latrines and keep hands, food, and kitchens clean.

OBJECTIVES for children's understanding and action

Children should:

● Understand that for babies and young children to grow strong, they need enough of the right kind of food and to eat frequently.

● Understand that babies and young children need to eat frequently because their stomachs are much smaller than those of adults.

● Understand that babies are well and healthy if they gain weight regularly.

● Understand that it is important to weigh babies regularly and know how to keep records to check that they are gaining weight.

● Know how to measure height and weight of themselves and other children.

● Know how to recognize children who are too thin, and some reasons why children might be thin.

● Know how to help children who have been ill by giving them extra meals.

UNDERSTANDING about child growth

1. Keeping a record of our growth

- **Children keep a scrapbook on 'Growing up'**

In it, they note how their height changes, what happens to their teeth, the size of their shoes, how their likes and dislikes change, how their faces change, and any other changes in their appearance.

- **Make a height measure in the classroom**

Mark 10 centimetre intervals on the wall, or on a door or window frame. (If one centimetre intervals are not marked, these can be measured with a ruler.)

Children measure their heights against it. They do this regularly, perhaps every month or two. Help them to keep a proper record in their 'Growing up' books. Older children can plot a graph.

If possible, keep a record of weight as well. (This depends on the availability of scales.)

- **Discussion about different heights**
    - What are our ages?
    - How tall are our parents and grandparents?
    - Do most of us grow to the same height as our parents?
    - Are we quick growers or slow growers?
    - Have we been ill recently?
    - Are we eating enough good food?

2. Using and interpreting growth charts

- **Children study and learn how to use growth charts available to mothers through the Ministry of Health**

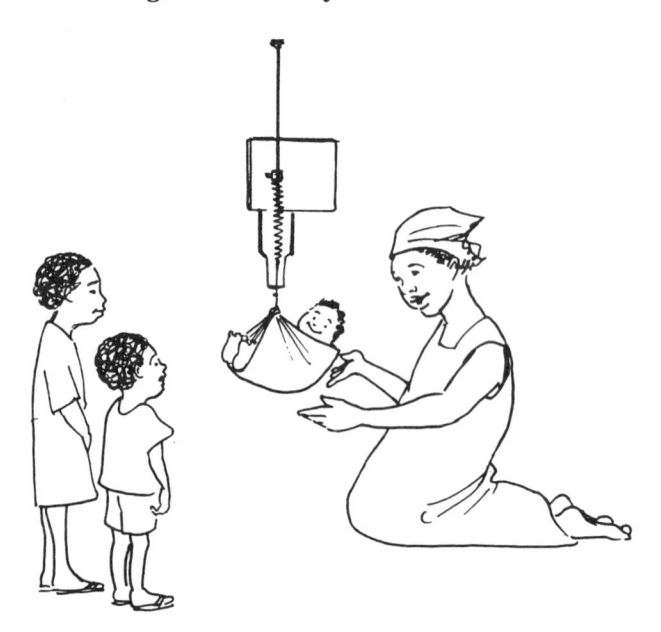

Health workers and teachers arrange for parents to bring babies into school so that children can watch them being weighed, and their weight recorded on the chart. The class takes a special interest in one baby and, with the agreement of the mother and father, the baby's growth chart is regularly brought in and discussed.

- **Older children learn to interpret the meaning of different dots and lines on the growth chart**

Here are the charts for three children and some examples of questions that can be asked:

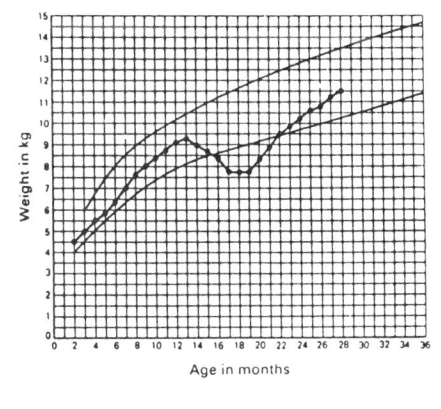

Miriam's chart

Raj's chart

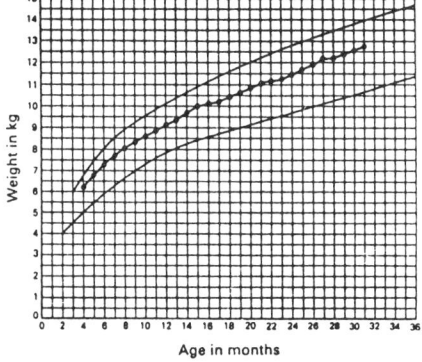

Musa's chart

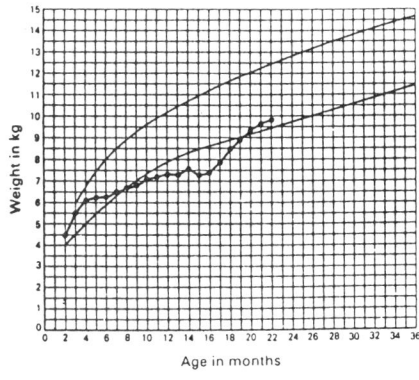

Sample questions:

☐ Which child has grown steadily?

☐ Which child lost weight after 13 months?

☐ Which child was ill after four months?

☐ When did Miriam start to get better?

☐ What weight was Raj at two years?

☐ When did Musa start to gain weight fast?

☐ How long did Miriam's illness last?

☐ What do you think Raj's weight might be by the time he is three years old if he continues to grow well?

3. Calculating how much and how often young children should eat

SMALL CHILDREN HAVE SMALL STOMACHS SO FEED THEM OFTEN!

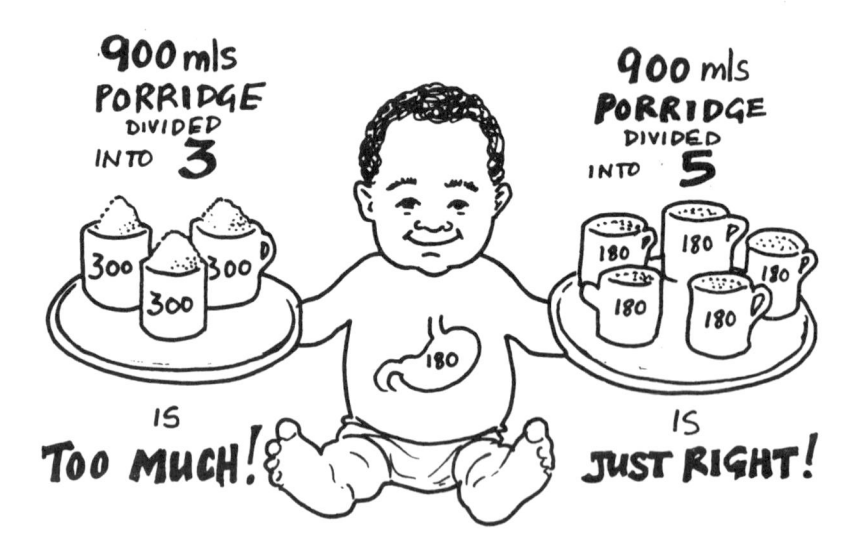

900 mls PORRIDGE DIVIDED INTO 3 — IS **TOO MUCH!**

900 mls PORRIDGE DIVIDED INTO 5 — IS **JUST RIGHT!**

- **Children calculate how many meals a young child needs**

The young child's stomach holds 180 ml.

The young child needs to eat 900 ml a day.

3 meals a day: 3 × 180 ml in the stomach = 540 ml.

4 meals a day: 4 × 180 ml in the stomach = 720 ml.

5 meals a day: 5 × 180 ml in the stomach = 900 ml.

Demonstrate this practically, using a small cup to represent a child's stomach and a bowl (about five times larger) to represent the food a child needs every day.

- **Children find out and record which oils and fats are locally available for cooking**

Oils used in cooking add calories without adding volume. Ask children how much oils and fats cost. Are some cheaper than others?

4. Children who are too thin ... a game to make children think

Often we accept very simple answers to the complex questions of health and development, e.g. children are too thin because they do not eat the right foods.

Yet it is important for children to understand that conditions such as malnutrition have many related causes.

Discuss with children whether they know any children who are 'too thin', and how to recognize signs of malnutrition. Then show a drawing of an imaginary child, 'Pedro', and ask, 'Why is Pedro so thin?' Each child suggests a different answer, for example, 'He does not get enough to eat'; 'His family is poor'; 'He has been ill'; 'The rains didn't come'.

The children begin to think of who could help Pedro and how. What action can be taken by his family, the community, and the government? What can children do? Children list ways in which they can help Pedro.

CHILDREN'S ACTION

I Can

- Help to record the weight of a baby at home.

    Children with small babies at home are asked to:
    - Find out whether the baby is weighed regularly and the weight recorded on a growth chart. (Children may be able to help mothers to get a growth chart.)
    - Help every time the baby is weighed and fill in the chart with mother (usually at the clinic).
    - Help explain the meaning of the growth chart when this is necessary, e.g. to father, aunt, childminder.
- Help mother to feed the baby.
- Help to feed my brother or sister after they have been ill. Explain to others at home why this is important.
- Look after the other children while mother takes the baby to the clinic.
- Measure the heights of younger brothers and sisters at home by marking heights on a wall (with name and date).

We Can

- Organize a 'better food' fair based on the school:

    - Give cooking demonstrations, especially of food for growth (*see pages 63 and 64 for ideas*, e.g. porridge enriched with mashed vegetables and a little oil or fat).

    - Show results of a poster competition.

    - Put on plays and puppet shows about feeding children often.

    - Have games and sideshows about feeding and growth for young children.
    (Many other activities are possible. Once a child-led committee is established, they will identify and plan activities themselves.)

- Have partners in the youngest class in the school and measure their heights regularly.

BASKET OF IDEAS

- Children visit the health worker who can tell them how families are advised about good feeding.

- Children learn how health workers recognize malnutrition by measuring mid-arm circumference of children between one and five years.

- Children find out how mothers in their community know when their babies are getting thinner. Some mothers put strings around the babies' arms, legs or hips. These strings need changing as the baby grows.

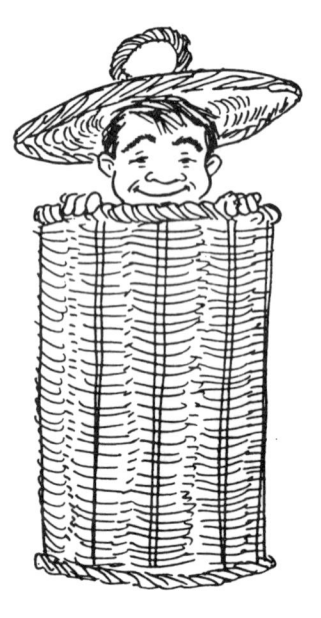

- Children make up a drama or a puppet show about two families, one with children who are growing well and one with children who are not. Why is this so? What can the families do? Can they help each other?

- Children make up songs about normal weight gain (e.g. a baby who is growing well doubles its birth weight by about five to six months).

EVALUATION QUESTIONS

Children
- Do we know our own height (and weight, if scales are available)?
- Have we measured the heights of our younger sisters and brothers?
- Can we fill in the growth chart?
- Have we been to the clinic to see how babies are weighed?
- Have we helped to give babies and young children four or five meals a day?
- Have we helped brothers and sisters who have been ill by encouraging them to eat an extra meal each day?

Teachers
Do children understand:
- The meaning of a growth chart?
- Why it is important to weigh babies monthly?
- The different reasons why some children are too thin?

Health Workers
- Have we helped children understand the importance of weighing babies and filling in the growth charts?

What children need to know and pass on about
Child Development

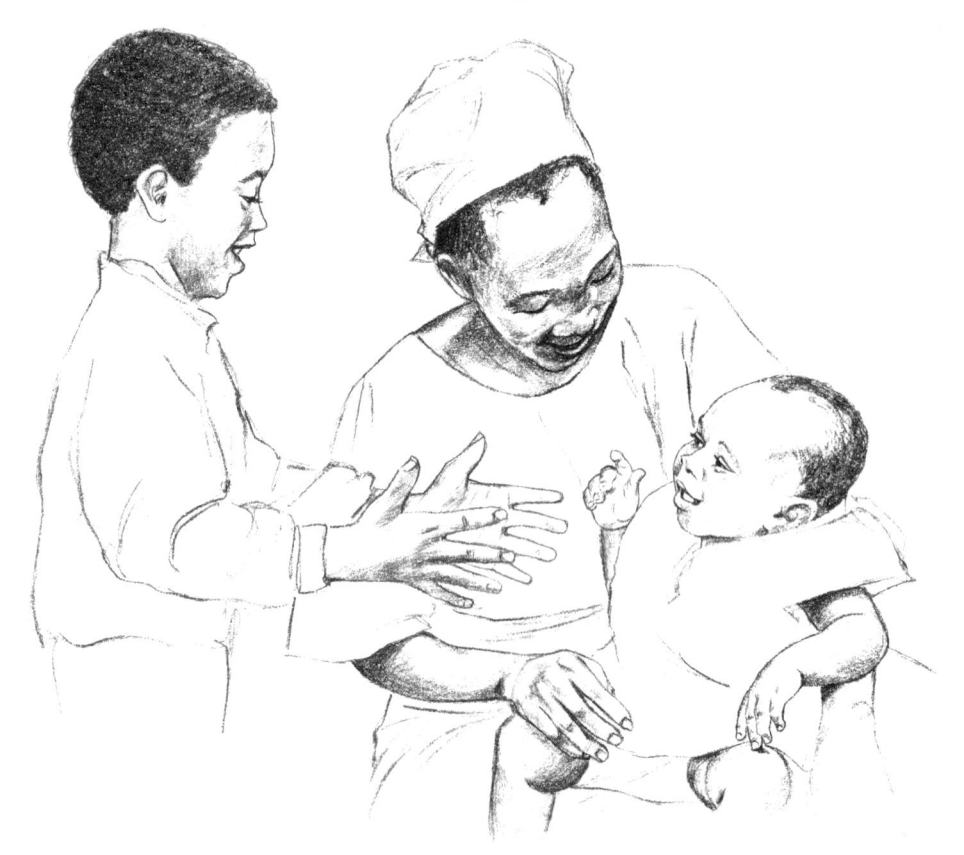

Everyone who loves, cares, and plays with babies can help them to learn and develop. Children, who spend so much time with their brothers and sisters, are among their most important 'teachers'.

The seven prime messages in this chapter can assist older children, together with their parents, to help young children grow up bright and happy – and to build the foundations for them to learn well at school.

PRIME MESSAGES
and supporting information

1 Babies begin to learn rapidly from the moment they are born. By age two, most of the growth of the human brain is already complete. For good mental growth, the child's greatest need is the love and attention of adults.

● A baby's five senses – sight, smell, hearing, taste, touch – are all working from the moment of birth. And from the moment of birth, a baby begins learning about the world.

● From birth, one of the greatest needs of all children is to be talked to, touched, cuddled, hugged, to see familiar faces and expressions and to hear familiar voices, and to see that others will respond to them. Children also need new and interesting things to look at, listen to, watch, hold, and play with. This is the beginning of learning. Human voices are the most important thing for the baby to hear. Human faces are the most important thing for the baby to see. Babies should not be left on their own for long periods of time.

● If a child has plenty of love and attention, and babyish play, as well as good nutrition and health care, then the child's mind will also grow well.

2 Play is important to a child's development. By playing, a child exercises mind and body, and absorbs basic lessons about the world. Parents can help a child to play.

● Children play because it is fun. But it is now known that play is also an important part of a child's development.

● By playing with simple objects and imitating the world of adults, children begin to learn about the world around them. Play also helps develop the skills of language, thinking, and organizing.
   Children learn by trying things out, comparing the results, asking questions, setting themselves new challenges, and finding ways to succeed. Play builds knowledge and experience, and helps a child to grow in curiosity, confidence, and control.

● Parents can help a child's play – and learning – by providing things to play with and suggesting new things for the child to try to do. But parents should not control or dominate the child's play too much. They should watch closely and follow the child's ideas and wishes.

Parents can help a child to do what he or she wants to do; but if parents do too much then the child loses the chance to learn by trying to do things for himself or herself. Children learn most from trying to do something and failing and then trying a different way and succeeding.

● When a very young child insists on trying to do something for himself or herself, parents should be patient. As long as the child is protected from danger, struggling to do something new and difficult is a necessary step in the child's development – even if it means some frustration. A little bit of frustration helps a child to learn and master new skills. Too much frustration can be discouraging and gives the child a sense of failure. Parents are the best judge of when to offer help and when to leave children to find their own solutions.

● Children love to dress up and pretend to be someone else – mother, father, teacher, doctor, or some imaginary character. This kind of play is also important. It helps the child to understand and accept the ways in which other people behave. It also helps to develop the child's imagination. Parents can encourage these 'let's pretend' games by giving children old clothes, hats, bags, beads, or pieces of fabric to play with and dress up in.

● Children sometimes need to play alone. But sometimes they need to play with adults as well. Talking to infants, repeating words and sounds, singing, music, nursery rhymes, repetitive babyish games – all of these are vital to the child's happiness and normal growth and development.

3 Children learn how to behave by imitating the behaviour of those closest to them.

● The example set by adults and older children is more powerful than words or 'orders' in shaping the growing child's behaviour and personality. If adults show their anger by shouting, aggression, and violence, children will learn that this is the right way to behave. If adults treat children and others with kindness, consideration, and patience, children will follow their example.

● Children under the age of about four years are naturally self-centred. Only gradually do they learn to share and consider others.

Selfish and unreasonable behaviour is normal in young children because they are emotionally as well as physically immature. As they grow up, children will learn to be unselfish and reasonable if others are unselfish and reasonable with them. They will learn to treat others as they themselves have been treated.

4 | **Young children easily become angry, frightened, and tearful. Patience, understanding, and sympathy with the child's emotions will help the child to grow up happy, well balanced, and well behaved.**

- A child's emotions are very real and powerful, even if they sometimes seem unreasonable to adults. Children may be frightened of strangers, or of the dark, or they may be very upset and cry about something very small. Or they may become unreasonably frustrated and angry if they are unable to do something or if they are told they cannot have something they want.

  Parents need to understand and sympathize with the child's emotions. If crying or anger or fearfulness is laughed at or punished or ignored, children may grow up shy, withdrawn, and unable to express emotions in a normal way. If parents are patient and kind when a child is struggling with strong emotions, the child is more likely to grow up happy and well balanced.

- Young children sometimes appear to lie because they cannot yet tell the difference between the real world and the world of the imagination.

- When a child does something wrong or unacceptable, it should be pointed out firmly but calmly that this is not the way to behave. Simple and reasonable explanations should be given. Children remember explanations and rules given to them by adults whom they love and wish to please. Gradually they come to accept these examples and explanations as the basis for their own actions. It is in this way that the child comes to have a conscience and to understand the difference between right and wrong.

- Crying is a young child's way of saying that something is wrong. Maybe the child is hungry, or tired, or in pain or discomfort, or too hot or too cold, or has been startled, or needs to be held and cuddled. Crying should not be ignored.

- Some babies cry a lot and nothing seems to comfort them. Usually, this kind of crying begins at the age of three or four weeks and often happens at the same time each day. This may go on for up to three months. The cause of this kind of crying is not known. It does not seem to harm the child.

● Young children soon outgrow their fears if they have confidence that their home is safe and that they are loved and protected by their parents or other familiar adults.

5 · Children need frequent approval and encouragement. Physical punishment is bad for a child's development.

● If parents show approval of a child's behaviour, this encourages a child to be good. So it is important for parents to look out for good behaviour and to show their pleasure and approval. This is a much better way of teaching a child to behave than constant criticism, shouting, and punishment.

● Parents should show their delight when a child learns a new skill, however small. If the child receives no encouragement, or too much criticism, the desire to learn and develop new skills is reduced.

● Physical punishment is bad for children. It makes children more likely to grow up being unreasonable and violent towards others. It can also make children frightened, and this can destroy the child's natural desire to please and to learn from his or her parents and teachers.

6 · The foundations of learning well in school can be built by the parents in the earliest years of a child's life.

● In the earliest years of life, parents can help build the foundations for successful learning in school. From birth, a child who feels loved, secure, and approved of is more likely to have the desire and the confidence to learn rapidly.

Parents can also help a child to learn by playing. All children need simple play materials so that there is always something to do or to explore at each new stage of the child's development. This need not cost a lot of money. Water, sand, cardboard boxes, containers, wooden building blocks, safe household items, objects of different colours, a ball, and many traditional playthings are just as good as shop-bought toys. Whenever it is possible and safe, children should be allowed to make their own decisions. They learn best from their own successes and their own mistakes. Parents should try to guide but not control the child's play.

● Preschool and child-care programmes can help prepare a child to learn well at school – if they provide lots of care and attention and a variety of play activities to help a child develop skills.

● Too much pressure on a child to learn and to do well in school is not helpful. Teaching things like reading and writing and numbers at too early an age is like trying to build the top of a building first. Like a building, a child's capacity for learning grows in stages, each stage built upon the last. The child learns best if parents and school teachers provide the opportunity to learn whatever is appropriate at each stage. To do this requires skill and patience. It means watching very closely and knowing when a child is becoming too frustrated or too bored. And it means constantly providing new opportunities and just the right kind of new challenges and interests for the child to continue his or her own learning process.

● Learning to speak and understand language is one of the most important and complicated tasks facing young children. They learn best if parents are constantly helping, right from birth, by talking, singing songs and nursery rhymes, pointing at things or people and giving them names, asking questions, and reading or telling stories as soon as the child is able to understand. Children are able to understand language long before they can speak.

It is possible to have 'conversations' with a child from the very earliest age. It does not matter how simple or babyish the conversation is. What matters is 'bathing the child in words'. The child needs to respond to words and sounds and to see others respond to his or her own attempts at sounds and words. When a child begins to make sounds, words, and sentences, parents should show their delight and encourage the child to build on the things that have been learnt.

● Children learn to speak at different ages. In general, they begin to talk from about the age of one and can use complete sentences by the age of four. By age six, all the basics of language have usually been learnt. Encouragement and practice during these first six years is very important to the child's later success in learning to speak, read and write, and to do well at school.

● There is no difference between the physical, mental, and emotional needs of boy and girl children. Both have the same need for play and the same capacity for all kinds of learning – and both have the same need for expressions of love and approval.

7 | **A parent is the best observer of a child's development. So all parents should know the warning signs which mean that a child is not making normal progress and that something may be wrong.**

● Some children progress more slowly than others, and this in itself need not be a cause for alarm.

● The following is a parents' guide to what children should be able to do at three months, twelve months, two years, four years, and five years of age. If a child cannot do these things at the right age, this does not necessarily mean that there is a serious problem. But it does mean that the matter should be discussed with a health worker.

At three months, does your child:
Turn head towards bright colours and lights?
Move eyes to loud sounds?
Make fists with both hands?
Wiggle and kick with legs and arms?
Smile?
Make cooing sounds?

At twelve months, does your child:
Sit without support?
Crawl on hands and knees?
Get up to standing position (with support)?
Pick things up with thumb and one finger?
Follow simple directions?
Give affection?
Say two or three words?

At two years, does your child:
Use two- or three-word sentences?
Recognize familiar people and objects?
Carry an object while walking?
Repeat words that others say?
Feed himself or herself?
Identify hair, ears and nose by pointing?

At four years, does your child:
Balance on one foot?
Play simple games with others?
Ask questions?
Answer simple questions?
Show different emotions?
Wash hands alone?
Point to six basic colours?

At five years, does your child:
Speak clearly?
Dress without help?
Copy a circle, square, triangle?
Count five to ten objects?

OBJECTIVES for children's understanding and action

Children should:

● Understand that babies and young children pass through certain stages of development, e.g. learning to smile, sit, walk, talk.

● Understand that at each stage of development babies can be helped to learn. Playing and talking with babies helps them develop faster.

● Know how to encourage play, and make and use toys that help babies and young children to develop their curiosity and knowledge of the world around them.

● Understand that babies need love and attention for mental growth and that neglecting young children or treating them badly limits their development.

● Understand why young children may easily become angry, frightened or tearful.

UNDERSTANDING about child development

1. Making a record of baby's development

Baby's development card

Children mark a sheet of paper into 4 sections across and 13 sections down the page as is partly shown in the diagram. The sections across are the weeks in the month; 1, 2, 3 or 4. The sections down are the months 3-15. Label the sections 3 months, 4 months, 5 months, 6 months, etc. up to 15 months in the left hand side.

Each week children ask their mothers and write down the new things their own baby can do. They may like to decorate the card around the edges and take it home for their mother to hang it up for all the family to

Name:		Date of birth:	
Week 1	Week 2	Week 3	Week 4
Month 3 — Baby opens eyes when I clap	Baby grasps wooden brick	Baby finds his mouth with his thumb	
4		Baby takes bamboo ring to his mouth		
5 — Baby drops a brick and takes a second one		Baby makes cooing sounds	Baby puts toe in his mouth

Chart continues as baby develops

79

see. In school, they display it and explain to other children how they observed the exciting development of their baby brother or sister.

2. Looking at ourselves now ... how are we different from babies?

Children tell, then mime the stages they passed through from when they were very small until now.
First we ... (smiled)
Then we ... (sat up)
Then we ...
Then we ...

Other children (and the teacher) challenge the order or suggest what has been forgotten.

3. Recording songs and games

Children discuss what songs and games they know for playing with babies before they can walk and talk. They ask grandparents what songs and games they know.

List the songs and games under headings, e.g.:

☐ Lullabies.

☐ Songs with actions.

☐ Games using fingers and toes.

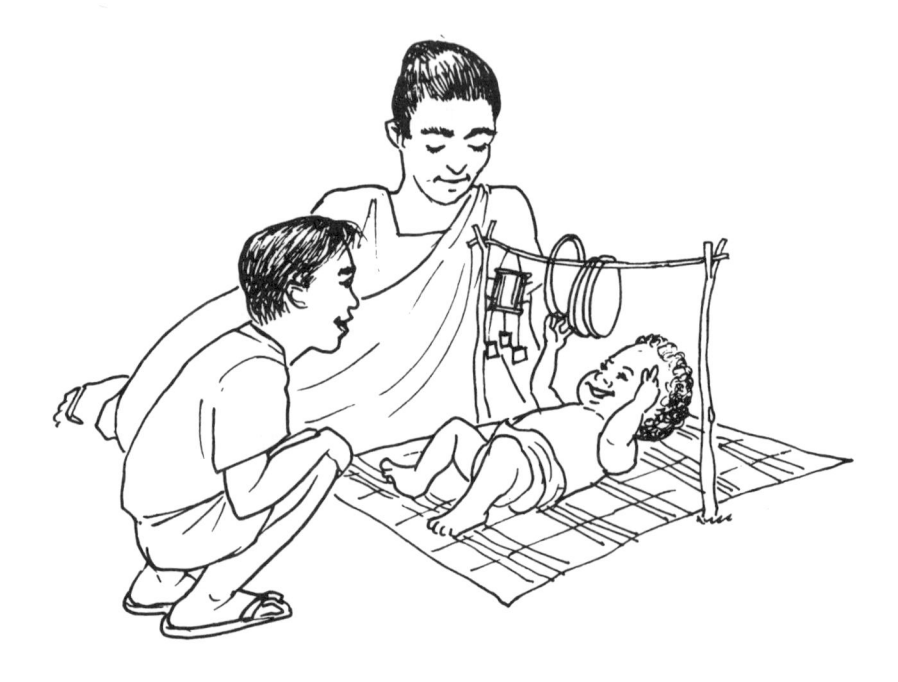

☐ Games using objects (like passing a small box or a soft ball from one hand to another).

☐ Action games (such as gently throwing baby into the air and catching her).

Children try out all the songs and games with babies at home. Which did they like best? Back in class, children make an illustrated class book of games for babies.

4. Understanding feelings

- **Stories ... when I was little**

Older children remember and tell stories about 'When I was little'. They describe what made them happy; what made them sad; what frightened them most ... why? They write down and illustrate the stories.

- **Observing and reporting from home**

What makes the baby happy? What makes the baby cry? What frightens the baby?

- **Imagining ... if I were one year old**

How big would the goat seem to be?
How big would the chair seem to be?
What would make me cry?

Children draw or write about what they imagine.

- **Miming and talking about feelings**

Children mime simple situations and show feelings. For example: A boy is lost. A girl has torn her new book. A child snatches something from another.

Other children watch and discuss how they would feel in that situation. Then they suggest how they can help.

CHILDREN'S ACTION

I Can

● Play with babies at home. Help them to smile and laugh; grasp and hold things; hide and find things; sit up, crawl and walk.

● Talk with babies, and sing to them. Help them look at and talk about objects and pictures they see.

● Encourage them to say more words. Make a list of the words that they learn.

● Make toys and books for babies.

We Can

● Make toys together:

A TOY-MAKING WORKSHOP IN A SCHOOL OR YOUTH GROUP

Children make:

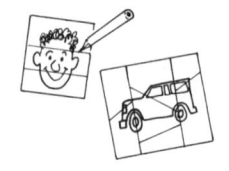

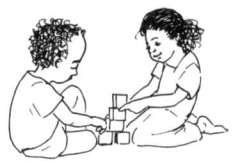

Play materials for building, sorting, fitting together

Play materials for imagination and pretending

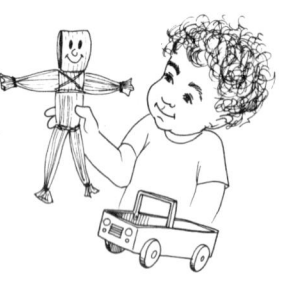

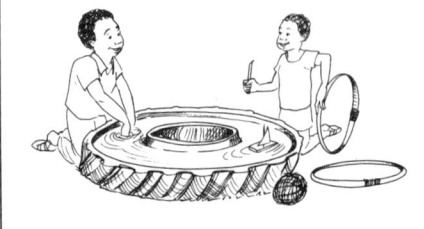

Play materials for outside games

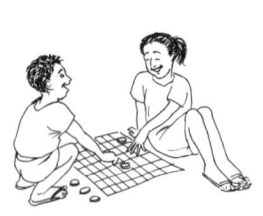

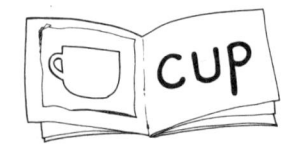

Play materials to start reading and counting

The toys and games that are made can be used by young children at home, in play groups and preschool groups, at the clinic waiting for treatment, or in hospital.

● Help to set up and organize safe places to play for ourselves and younger children.

● Watch over young children when they play.

BASKET OF IDEAS

● Older children give younger ones many different kinds of things to play with and sort: flowers with different colours and different smells; scraps of cloth which look and feel different; dull things and shiny things; big things and small things.

● Older children provide materials to help younger ones dress up and pretend. Paper, leaves, sticks and bits of cloth are used to make hats, dresses, and other 'pretend clothes'.

● Older children design games of throwing and catching, jumping and skipping, climbing and sliding, etc., that help younger children use the muscles in their bodies. What kinds of equipment do children need? What can this equipment be made from?

● Older children make simple drums and rattles, and teach younger ones to dance and sing, and play their instruments in time with songs.

● Older children provide materials that float and sink in water, or make water flow long distances. They make reed pipes of different sizes that water flows out of at different rates, or that are used for blowing bubbles. They collect containers of different shapes and sizes for younger ones to use when playing with water and mud.

● Older children collect scrap paper, cardboard, newspapers, etc., for young children to paint and draw on. They make paints from inks, dyes or local plants, and brushes from chewed sticks. They make glue from a local food like flour, mixed with a little water.

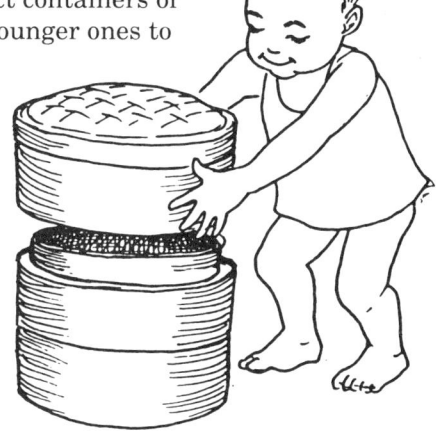

EVALUATION QUESTIONS

Children
- Are we playing with our baby more? differently?
- Who talks to the baby now? Is there a change?
- What toys have we made?
- What are the favourites?
- What games have we played?
- Are play areas well organized, safe, clean and tidy?

Teachers
- Is the school collecting waste/free materials for use in craft work, including toy-making?
- Are children helped or encouraged to make toys, either in class or out of class?
- Have children taught each other new songs and rhymes to sing with their younger brothers and sisters?
- Are children showing more sensitivity to each other's feelings (particularly older children to younger ones)?

Health Workers
- Have children made toys for babies and young children at the clinic?
- Do mothers at the clinic show more interest in children's play?

What children need to know and pass on about
Hygiene

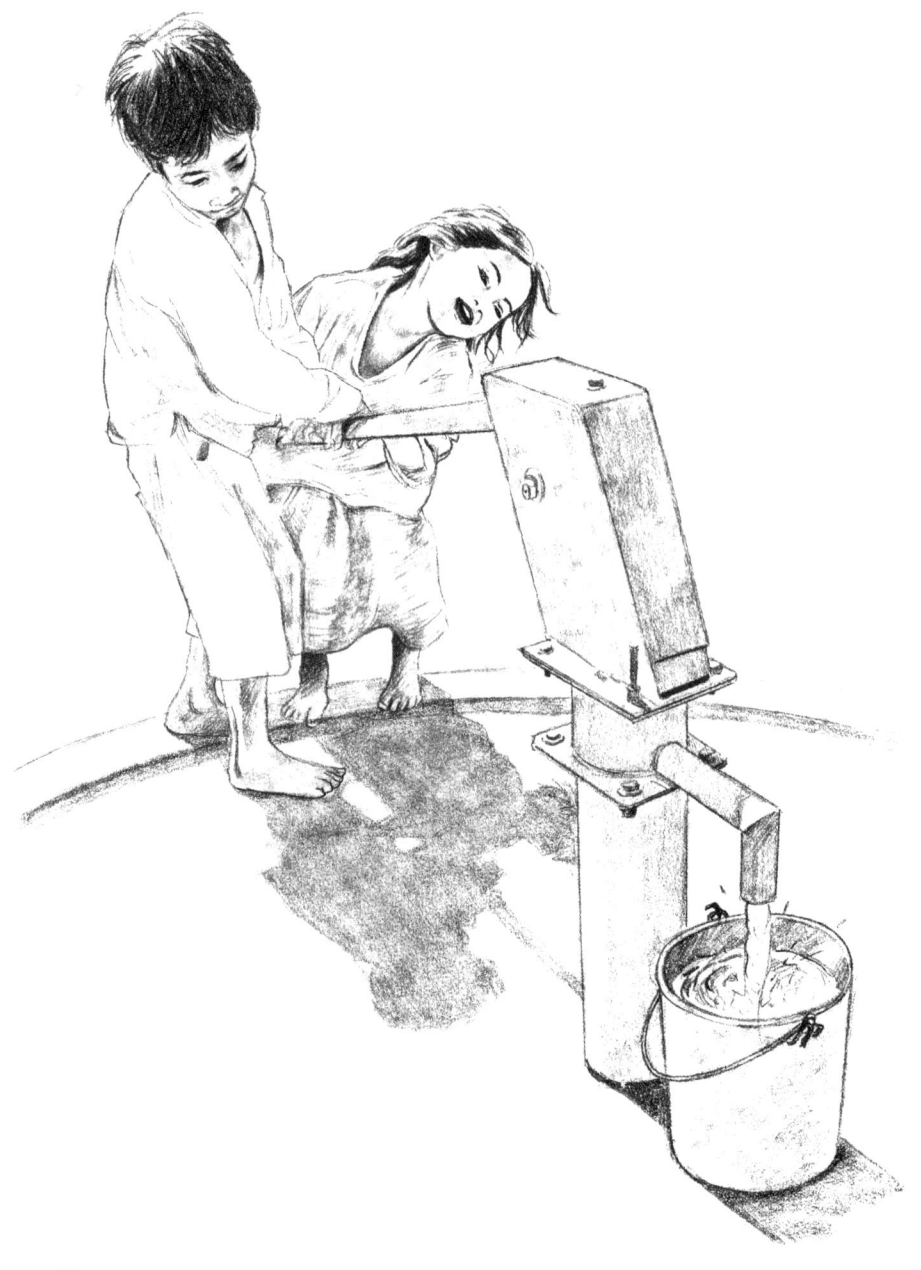

More than half of all illness and death among young children is caused by germs which get into the child's mouth via food and water. The seven prime messages of this chapter can help families and communities to prevent the spread of germs and so reduce illness and deaths.

It is important to stress that these messages, to be fully effective, must be acted upon by everyone in the community. Children have a particular part to play because of the care they provide for younger children and the example they can set for their peers and families.

In communities without latrines, without safe drinking water, and without safe refuse disposal, it is very difficult for families to prevent the spread of germs. It is therefore also vital for the government to support communities by providing – as a minimum – the materials and technical advice needed to construct latrines and improve drinking water supplies.

To demand such services, everyone in the community, including children, needs to know the facts about how illness is spread. Today's children are tomorrow's community leaders.

PRIME MESSAGES
and supporting information

1 Illnesses can be prevented by washing hands with soap and water after contact with faeces and before handling food.

● Washing hands with soap and water removes germs from the hands. This helps to stop germs from getting onto food or into the mouth. Soap and water should be easily available for all members of the family to wash their hands.

● It is especially important to wash hands after defecating, before handling food, and after cleaning the bottom of a baby or child who has just defecated. It is also important to wash hands after handling animals and after preparing raw foods.

● Children often put their hands into their mouths. So it is important to wash a child's hands often, especially before giving food.

● A child's face should be washed at least once every day. This helps to keep flies away from the face and to prevent eye infections. Soap is helpful for washing, but not absolutely essential.

2 | Illnesses can be prevented by using latrines.

● The single most important action that families can take to prevent the spread of germs is to dispose of faeces safely. Many illnesses, especially diarrhoea, come from the germs found in human faeces. People can swallow these germs if the germs get into water, onto food, onto the hands, or onto utensils and surfaces used for preparing food.

● To prevent this happening:

- Use latrines.
- If it is not possible to use a latrine, adults and children should defecate well away from houses, paths, water supplies, and anywhere that children play. After defecating, the faeces should be buried. Contrary to common belief, the faeces of babies and young children are even more dangerous than those of adults. So even small children should be taken to use the latrine. If children defecate without using a latrine, then their faeces should be cleared up immediately and put down the latrine or buried.
- Latrines should be cleaned regularly and kept covered.
- The faeces of animals should be kept away from homes and water sources.

3 | Illnesses can be prevented by using clean water.

● Families who have a plentiful supply of safe piped water, and know how to use it, have fewer illnesses.

● Families without a safe piped water supply can reduce illnesses if they protect their water supply from germs by:

- Keeping wells covered.
- Keeping faeces and waste water (especially from latrines) well away from any water used for cooking, drinking, bathing or washing.
- Keeping buckets, ropes and jars used to collect and store

water as clean as possible (for example by hanging up buckets rather than putting them on the ground).
- ☐ Keeping animals away from drinking water.
- Families can keep water clean in the home by:
  - ☐ Storing drinking water in a clean, covered container.
  - ☐ Taking water out of the container with a clean ladle or cup.
  - ☐ Not allowing anyone to put their hands into the container or to drink directly from it.
  - ☐ Keeping animals out of the house.

4 | **Illnesses can be prevented by boiling drinking water if it is not from a safe piped supply.**

- Even if water is clear, it may not be free from germs. The safest drinking water is from a piped supply. Water from other sources is more likely to contain germs.

- Boiling water kills germs. So, if possible, water drawn from sources such as ponds, streams, springs, wells, tanks, or public standpipes should be brought to the boil and cooled before drinking. It is especially important to boil and cool the water that is given to babies and young children; they have less resistance to germs than adults.

- If boiling or disinfecting water is not possible, it can be made safer by using sunlight. Choose containers made of colourless or light blue glass or plastic. You must be able to see through them. Remove all labels, fill with the cleanest water available, and cover the containers to keep out dirt and insects. Put them in an open space where the sun can shine on them all day. Spread them out so that they do not shade each other. Leave the containers in the sunlight for at least a day. The longer the containers are in sunlight, the greater the chance that the water will be safe. This method of making water safer does not work on cloudy days.

5 | **Raw food is often dangerous. It should be washed or cooked. Cooked food should be eaten straight away – not left to stand. Warmed-up food should be thoroughly reheated.**

- Thorough cooking kills germs. Food should be cooked right through – especially meat and poultry.

- Germs like warm food. Cooked food should be eaten as soon as possible after cooking so it does not have time to collect germs and cause illness.

- If food has to be kept for more than five hours, it should either be kept hot (above 60°c) or kept cooled (below 10°c).
- If cooked food is saved, it should be thoroughly reheated all the way through before being used again.
- Raw food, especially poultry, usually contains germs. Cooked food can be contaminated by even the slightest contact with raw food. So raw and cooked foods should always be kept away from each other. Knives, chopping boards, and food-preparing surfaces should always be cleaned after preparing raw food.
- Pasteurized or freshly boiled milk is safer than raw cow's milk.
- If possible, food prepared for infants should be freshly made and not stored.
- Cloths for cleaning dishes or pans should be changed every day if possible and boiled before being used again.

6 Illnesses can be prevented by keeping food clean.

● Germs on food can enter the body and cause illness. But food can be kept safe by:
- Keeping food-preparing surfaces clean. Germs grow in spots of dirt or food.
- Keeping food clean and covered and away from flies, rats, mice, dogs and other animals. Sealed containers are best.

7 Illnesses can be prevented by burning or burying household refuse.

● Germs can be spread by flies, which like to breed in refuse such as food scraps and peelings from fruit and vegetables. Every family should have a special pit where household refuse is buried or burned every day.

OBJECTIVES for children's understanding and action

Children should:

● Understand that many illnesses, including diarrhoea, worms and other intestinal parasites, result from poor hygiene and in particular from contamination of food and water by germs from hands infected by faeces.

● Understand that illnesses can be prevented by washing hands with soap and water after contact with faeces and before handling food.

● Understand why latrines must be built and used; and know how to keep them clean and safe.

● Understand that little children's faeces are especially dangerous; know how to get rid of faeces in a safe way; and how to train young children in cleaner habits.

● Know how to keep water clean and safe, both where it is found and when it is being stored and used.

● Know how food can be prepared and stored to make it safe to eat; and understand the importance of washing utensils for cooking and eating, to remove all traces of food.

● Understand that flies spread germs; know where flies breed; and how to prevent illness by burying or burning refuse (rubbish).

UNDERSTANDING about hygiene

1. Pictures to promote discussion of how faeces spread disease

With the help of a picture or blackboard drawing, hold a class discussion about ways in which faeces spread disease.

In groups of eight to 10, each child then draws a picture to show how faeces of children, adults and animals spread disease. Children in the group look at the pictures, and discuss and list the dangers. They make an oral report to the whole class.

Afterwards each child draws a second picture of how the disease could be prevented by better hygiene.

2. A survey ... where and how do we get our water?

Help children do a simple survey to find out for themselves that:

  □ There may be different water sources with varying water quality used for different purposes, e.g. washing clothes, drinking.

  □ Everyone in the community can affect water quality by their actions, such as covering wells and protecting the surroundings from cattle.

Help children to organize their work in six stages:

One

Let's find out the answers to these questions:

- Where are the different water sources in the area?
- How much water is provided in each place?
- How clear is the water?
- What are the surroundings like in each place – at the well, the stream, the tap?
- How is the water source protected?
- How could it be contaminated?
- How do we carry our water?
- How long does it take to walk home?

Two

How will we collect the information?

- Each child reports on the water source the family use, answering the questions above, OR
- Older pupils divide into groups and each group visits one or two sources, OR
- If the sites are quite close, the whole class visits the sources.

Three

How will we make a record of the information?

- Make a table with the water sources along the top, and the questions down the side. Fill in the answers across the page.

Four

How will we display the information?

- Make a big map of the area, with each water source shown and comments next to it.
- Children draw the container used in their family to fetch water, cut round the drawing and fix it alongside their water source.
- They mark the approximate position of their house on the map.

Five

What can we learn from the information?

- The number of sources of water available in the wet and dry seasons.
- The number of families in the class using each source.

- The quality of water at each source.
- The water sources which need community action to improve them.
- Who collects water and how much time it takes.
- If people did not have to collect water, how might the time saved be used to improve health?

Six

How can we use the information?
- To show which water sources need improvement.
- To encourage community action.

3. An experiment and demonstration ... how latrines can pollute water supplies

Help children choose a large container and fill it with sand. Sprinkle plenty of water on the sand. The water will collect at the bottom and form an underground pool equivalent to the 'water table' from which wells draw their water. Stick a cylinder pierced with small holes in the sand (use half a plastic bottle without a base), removing sand as necessary. This represents a well. Water will rise in it. Stick another, smaller cylinder close to the well. This is the latrine. Pour a coloured liquid such as ink or dye into the latrine. This represents urine and faeces. The dye will reach the underground pool and colour the water. After a while the water in the well with also be coloured.

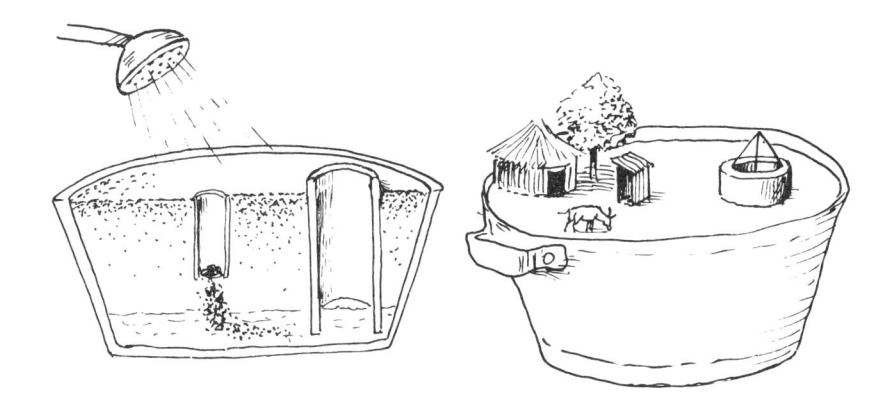

Ask children to:
- Draw and write about the experiment.
- Explain it to another class.

4. Looking at dirty water from a pond

Borrow a lens, or better still a microscope, from the local secondary school, to see the tiny organisms swimming about. Some of these are harmful (the germs). Boiling water kills most of these germs, but placing it in sunlight, in a clear glass or plastic bottle, also kills germs. Filtering water is another way of making it safer to drink.

5. Model-making ... dirty flies

Children make large model flies using available materials such as seeds, clay, six bent twig legs and two leaf wings.

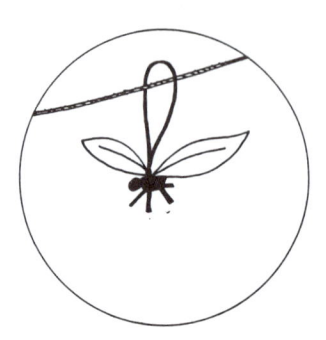

Other children make models or pictures of food for the flies to 'walk' on (or use real food).

The flies are made to 'walk' in dirt and then on a clean surface. This shows how they spread germs on their feet.

Hang some of the flies on a sloping string across the classroom to show how flies pass from a picture of human or animal faeces to a picture of food on a plate.

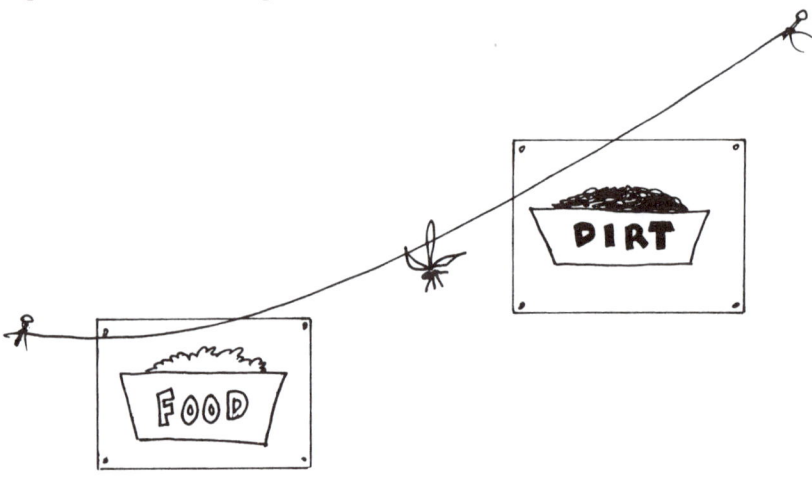

6. Stories and drama ... action to improve hygiene

Children write stories and then act them. Here are some ideas to help children start their stories. Discuss these story beginnings with children and then let them develop them in their own way. Pairs of children can co-operate in writing stories. The best stories can be dramatized.

The Water Dirtiers

☐ *Some powerful and selfish people in the community make the village water source dirty with their animals or by throwing rubbish in it ...*

(What can children do? How can they get help from older people in the village?)

My Life as a Fly

☐ *I'm Filthy the Fly and I have a sad story to tell you. I was living very happily with all my family and friends in a house. The people who lived there understood our habits very well. They never covered their food; they never covered the latrine; and they always kept their rubbish very near the house.*

But then, one day, their children came home from school. We hate these children ...

(Go on to say how the children drove the flies away from the house.)

My Little Sister

☐ *My little sister started to walk when she was 11 months old. Soon she was running all round the house, but of course her bottom wasn't clean and she made messes on the floor.*

'Don't worry,' said my uncle, 'she's only a little child and it isn't really dirty – just clean up the floor.'

I wasn't sure that he was right. I went to see my cousin who is a health worker ...

(The cousin tells the child that little children's faeces spread disease. What can the child do to convince her uncle?)

CHILDREN'S ACTION

I Can

● Take little brothers and sisters to the latrine, or cover or bury their faeces.

● Never urinate in water or pass faeces near water; and tell other children not to do so.

● Always wash my hands after using the latrine and before eating, and help little children do the same.

● Keep animals out of the house.

● Keep the water container in my house clean and covered, and always use a scoop.

● Make and use fly swats to kill flies.

We Can

● Form a school health committee to improve our school hygiene.

A SCHOOL HEALTH COMMITTEE

The committee is made up of elected representatives from each class, advised by a teacher and/or parent, e.g. a nurse.

The committee should:

● Make a set of school hygiene rules and display them.

● Arrange, where possible, for clean drinking water in each class; and for washing water near the latrine, and the kitchen if food is prepared in school.

● Help organize children to keep their classrooms and surroundings clean.

● Monitor the latrines, and check that they are covered and kept as clean as possible.

● Arrange for older children to assist young ones with their hygiene.

● Organize plays, talks and puppet shows for the rest of the school.

● Survey the food-sellers near the school. Buy from those who sell fresh food and keep it clean.

● Make a village health map or model. Display the map or model at a school open day and explain it to visitors.

● Make and use crafts such as food safes and covers, latrine covers, water filters and water pot scoops.

● Take action to keep wells clean; make a stand to keep the container and rope off the ground. Make a small wall round the well to keep animals away and prevent water that is spilt running back into the well.

● Write to the neighbourhood council suggesting why we think the water supply needs to be improved (based on our survey – *see pages 91-93*).

VILLAGE HEALTH MAP

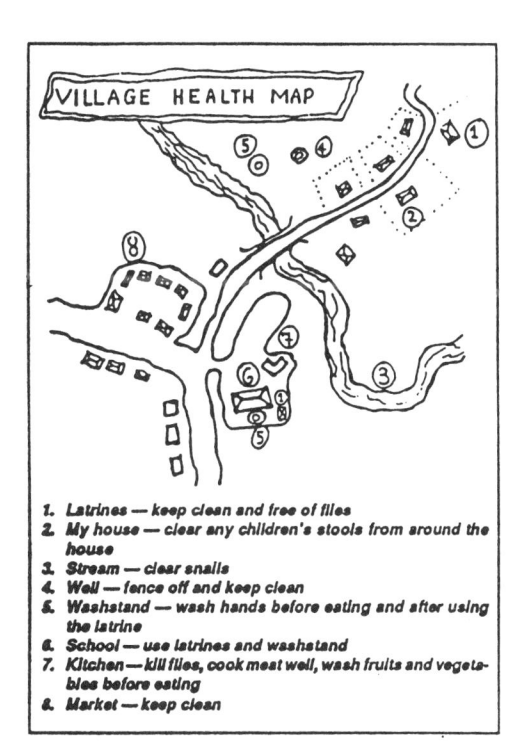

1. *Latrines — keep clean and free of flies*
2. *My house — clear any children's stools from around the house*
3. *Stream — clear snails*
4. *Well — fence off and keep clean*
5. *Washstand — wash hands before eating and after using the latrine*
6. *School — use latrines and washstand*
7. *Kitchen — kill flies, cook meat well, wash fruits and vegetables before eating*
8. *Market — keep clean*

BASKET OF IDEAS

● Children carry out a home survey: how do we store water? how do we prevent people from contaminating the water with their hands when they get a drink?

● Children put out two plates, one with fresh food and one with rotten food. Observe what flies do.

● Older children watch a young child for a while and count how many times fingers, or an object, are placed in the mouth.

● Children make a series of pictures or a chart showing how water gets from the source to a drink at home.

● Older children learn or write songs about personal hygiene and teach them to little children.

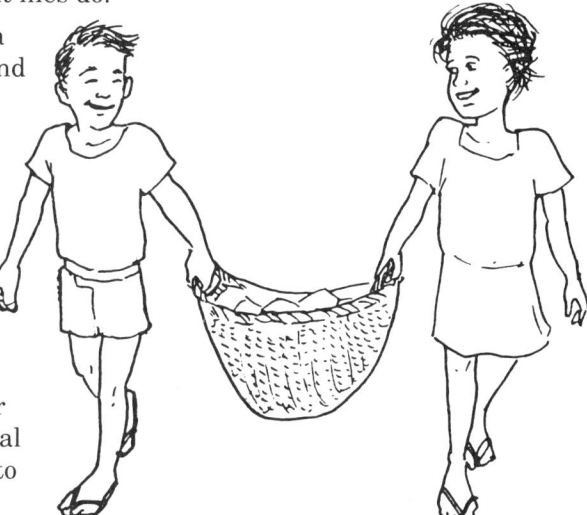

97

EVALUATION QUESTIONS

Children
- Do I use a latrine, or bury my faeces?
- Do I wash my hands after defecating?
- Do I wash my hands before eating?
- Do I have short, clean fingernails?
- Have I helped younger brothers and sisters to use a latrine or bury/cover their faeces?
- Have I helped younger children to wash their hands?
- Have I made a cover to keep flies off food and drink?
- Have I made and used a fly swat?

Teachers
- Have the children kept the school surroundings clean and attractive?
- Have they helped to keep the latrines clean?
- Have they organized a school health committee?
- Have they made and displayed posters about keeping water clean?
- Have they dug a pit for rubbish in the school compound and/or made rubbish bins from local materials?

Health Workers
- Have children helped in any way to improve community hygiene, including water supplies?

What children need to know and pass on about Diarrhoea

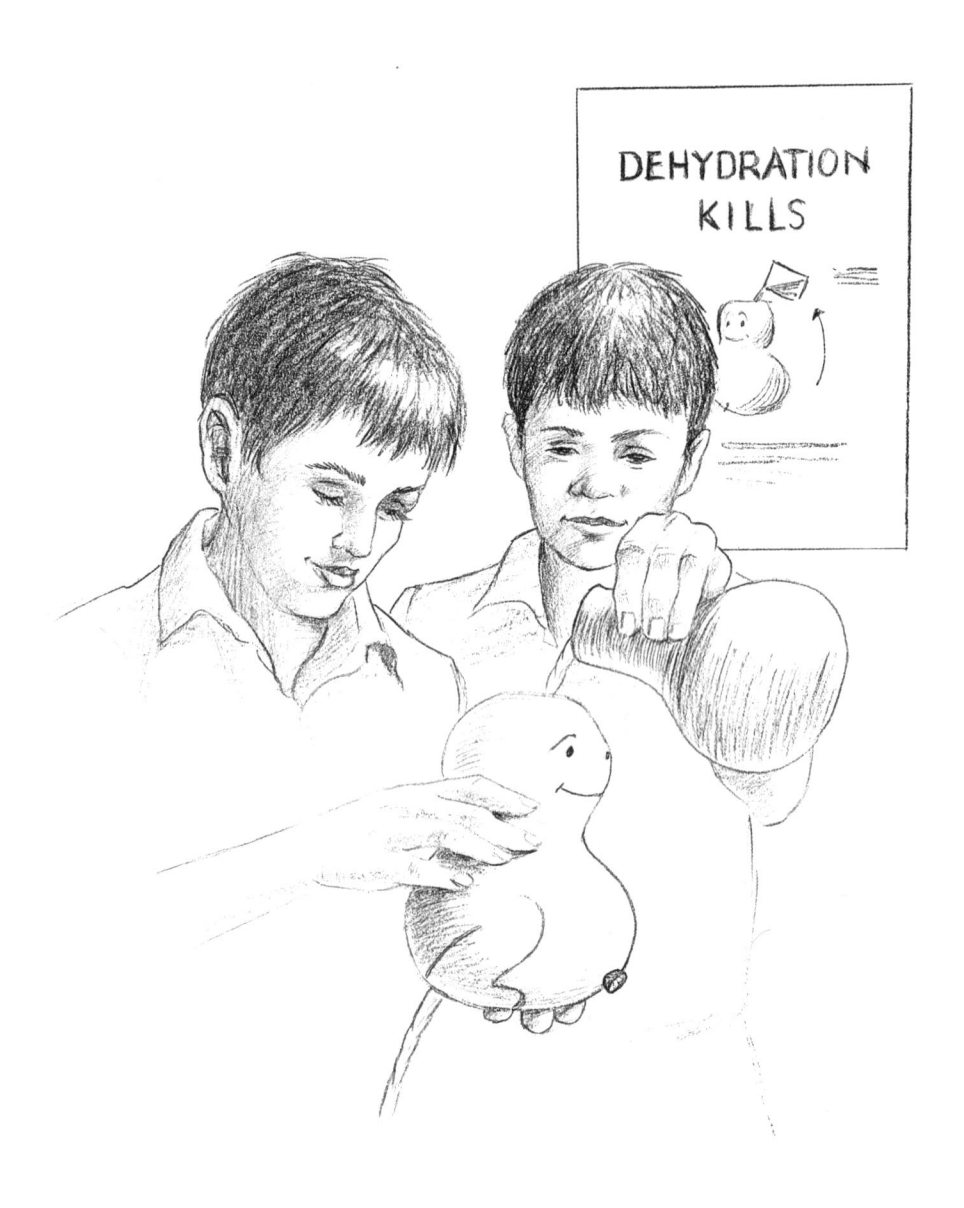

Using the gourd doll to demonstrate dehydration

Diarrhoea causes dehydration and malnutrition, and kills over three million children every year. Nearly all these deaths can be prevented and children helped to grow and develop.

The main causes of diarrhoea are poor hygiene, lack of clean drinking water, overcrowding, and the trend towards bottle-feeding rather than breastfeeding. It is the responsibility of government to support the community in tackling these basic problems.

Older children have a key role, both as family members and as future parents, in understanding the dangers of dehydration and learning to take action to prevent it at home. They can recognize when dehydration is severe and needs medical help. They are also powerful agents in spreading messages concerning the importance of feeding younger children with diarrhoea.

PRIME MESSAGES
and supporting information

1 Diarrhoea can kill children by draining too much liquid from the body. So it is essential to give a child with diarrhoea plenty of liquids to drink.

● Diarrhoea is dangerous. Roughly one in every two hundred children who get diarrhoea will die from it.

● Most often, diarrhoea kills by dehydration. This means that too much liquid has been drained out of the child's body. So as soon as diarrhoea starts, it is essential to give the child extra drinks to replace the liquid being lost.

● Suitable drinks to prevent a child from losing too much liquid during diarrhoea are:

   ☐ Breastmilk.
   ☐ Gruels (mixtures of cooked cereals and water).
   ☐ Soups.
   ☐ Rice water.
   ☐ Fresh fruit juices.

- Weak teas.
- Green coconut water.
- Water from the cleanest possible source (if possible, brought to the boil and then cooled).
- Oral rehydration salts solution.

● In almost all countries, special drinks for children with diarrhoea are available in pharmacies, shops, or health centres. Usually, these come in the form of packets of oral rehydration salts (ORS) to be mixed with the recommended amount of clean water (*see box on next page*). Although ORS is especially made for the treatment of dehydration, it can also be used to prevent dehydration.

Do not add ORS to liquids such as milk, soup, fruit juice or soft drinks.

● If ORS is not available, dehydration can be treated by giving the child a drink made from four level teaspoons of sugar and half a level teaspoon of salt dissolved in one litre of clean water.

This is less salt and less sugar than recommended in the first edition of *Facts for Life*. In practice, too much salt and sugar have sometimes been used because spoon sizes differ and because parents sometimes add more salt and sugar in the belief that this will make the treatment more effective. But too much sugar can make the diarrhoea worse and too much salt can be harmful to the child. Therefore a more dilute formula is now recommended. If the mixture is made a little too dilute, no harm can be done, and there is very little loss of effectiveness.

● To replace the liquid being lost from the child's body, one of these drinks should be given to the child every time a watery stool is passed:

- Between a quarter and a half of a large cup for a child under the age of two.
- Between a half and a whole large cup for older children.

● The drink should be given directly from a cup or by a teaspoon – not from a feeding bottle. If the child vomits, wait for 10 minutes and then begin again, giving the drink to the child slowly, small sips at a time.

● Extra liquids should be given until the diarrhoea has stopped. This will usually take between three and five days.

ORS – a special drink

A special drink for diarrhoea can be made by using a packet of oral rehydration salts (ORS). This drink is used by doctors and health workers to treat dehydrated children. But it can also be used in the home to prevent dehydration.

- Dissolve the contents of the packet in the amount of water indicated on the packet. If you use too little water, the drink could make the diarrhoea worse. If you use too much water, the drink will be less effective.
- Stir well, and give to the child to drink in a cup or feed with a spoon.

2 | A child with diarrhoea needs food.

● It is often said that a child with diarrhoea should not be given any food or drink while the diarrhoea lasts. This advice is wrong. Food can help to stop the diarrhoea. Also, diarrhoea can lead to serious malnutrition unless parents make a special effort to keep feeding the child during and after the illness.

● A child with diarrhoea usually has less appetite, so feeding may be difficult at first. But the child should be tempted to eat – as frequently as possible – by offering small amounts of his or her favourite foods.

● After the age of about six months, all children need extra food in addition to breastmilk. They should be given soft, well-mashed mixes of cereal and beans, or cereal and well-cooked meat or fish. Add one or two teaspoonfuls of oil to cereal and vegetable mixes if possible. Also good for the child are yoghurt and fruits. Foods should be freshly prepared and given to the child five or six times a day. This diet should be continued if the child has diarrhoea.

3 | When a breastfed child has diarrhoea, it is important to continue breastfeeding.

● Mothers are sometimes advised to give less breastmilk if a child has diarrhoea. This is wrong advice. Breastfeeding should continue – and if possible the child should be fed more often.

● If the child is being fed on milk-powder solutions or cow's milk, then feeding should continue as usual.

4 | A child who is recovering from diarrhoea needs an extra meal every day for at least two weeks.

● Extra feeding after the diarrhoea stops is vital for a full recovery. At this time, the child has more appetite and can eat an extra meal a day for at least two weeks. This will help the child to catch up on the food 'lost' while the child was ill and the appetite was low. A child is not fully recovered from diarrhoea until he or she is at least the same weight as when the illness began.

● Breastfeeding more frequently than usual also helps to speed up recovery.

5 | Trained help is needed if diarrhoea is more serious than usual, if it persists for more than two weeks, or if there is blood in the stool.

● Parents should seek help from a health worker without delay if the child:
- Has a fever.
- Is extremely thirsty.
- Will not eat or drink normally.
- Vomits frequently.
- Passes several watery stools in one or two hours.
- Passes blood in the stool (a sign of dysentery).

or:
- If the diarrhoea persists for more than two weeks.

● If a child has any of these signs, qualified medical help is needed quickly. The doctor or health worker will give the child a drink made with special oral rehydration salts (*see box page 103*). In the meantime, keep trying to make the child drink liquids.

6 | Medicines other than ORS should not be used for diarrhoea, except on medical advice.

● Most medicines for diarrhoea are either useless or harmful. The diarrhoea will usually cure itself in a few days. The real danger is usually not the diarrhoea but malnutrition and the loss of liquids from the child's body.

● Do not give a child tablets or other medicines for diarrhoea unless these have been prescribed by a trained health worker.

● Antibiotics should be given – after seeking medical advice – if a child has diarrhoea with blood in the stool. Other drugs should not be used.

7 | **Diarrhoea can be prevented by breastfeeding, by immunizing all children against measles, by using latrines, by keeping food and water clean, and by washing hands before touching food.**

● Diarrhoea is caused by germs from faeces entering the mouth. These germs can be spread in water, in food, on hands, on eating and drinking utensils, by flies, and by dirt under fingernails. To prevent diarrhoea, the germs must be stopped from entering the child's mouth.

● Poverty and lack of basic services such as clean drinking water mean that many families find it difficult to prevent diarrhoea. But the most effective ways are to:

- Give breastmilk alone for about the first six months of a baby's life (breastmilk helps to protect babies against diarrhoea and other illnesses).

- At the age of about six months, introduce clean, nutritious, well-mashed, semi-solid foods and continue to breastfeed.

- If a milk-powder solution or cow's milk has to be used, give it to the child from a cup rather than a bottle.

- Use the cleanest water available for drinking (water from wells, springs or rivers should be brought to the boil and cooled before use).

- Always use latrines to dispose of faeces, and be sure to put children's faeces in a latrine immediately (or bury them). (Children's faeces are even more dangerous to health than those of adults.)

- Wash hands with soap and water immediately after using the latrine and before preparing or eating food.

- Cover food and drinking water to protect it from germs.

- If possible, food should be thoroughly cooked, and prepared just before eating. It should not be left standing, or it will collect germs.

- Bury or burn all refuse to stop flies spreading disease.

● Measles frequently results in serious diarrhoea. Immunization against measles therefore also protects a child against this cause of diarrhoea. There is no vaccine to prevent ordinary diarrhoea.

OBJECTIVES for children's understanding and action

Children should:

● Understand what is meant by diarrhoea and dehydration; and that diarrhoea can kill, rapidly through dehydration or later because it causes malnutrition and weakens a child's resistance to disease.

● Know how to recognize the signs of diarrhoea and dehydration, especially the danger signs in severe diarrhoea which needs immediate treatment by a health worker.

● Understand the causes of diarrhoea, and especially the link between poor hygiene and diarrhoea.

● Know how diarrhoea is commonly treated in the community, and whether such treatments effectively prevent dehydration.

● Know how to make appropriate drinks and when to give them to children with diarrhoea.

● Understand that a child needs food as well as drink during and after diarrhoea; and that babies with diarrhoea should continue to be breastfed.

UNDERSTANDING about diarrhoea

1. A discussion ... what is diarrhoea and what causes it?

Start off with children's own experience. Describe the symptoms of diarrhoea and ask children:

- Who has been ill like this?
- When did you last have it?
- What do you call it at home?
- Has anyone heard the word 'diarrhoea'?

Base the discussion around key questions – not too many – such as:

- How do you recognize diarrhoea?
- Is diarrhoea just a nasty thing to have, or is it dangerous?
- Which age group gets it more often and why?
- Is there a particular time of the year when you and people in your family more often have diarrhoea? Do you know why?
- Are babies more likely to get it if they are fed with a bottle or if their mother breastfeeds them? Do you know why?

Follow the discussion with a summary of the main points learnt about diarrhoea.

2. A survey ... diarrhoea in our community

Help the children do a simple survey to find out for themselves:
- How common diarrhoea is in their community.
- That it is most common among children under five, particularly bottle-fed babies and babies who have started to eat other foods in addition to breastmilk.
- That it is most common in rainy seasons.
- That it may lead to dehydration and death.

Children organize their work on this survey in five stages:

One

Let's find out answers to these questions:
- Which children have had diarrhoea (either looking at the whole school, or at just one household)?
- Which age group has had it most often?
- Is there a season in which it is most common for children to get diarrhoea?
- Are there any babies or children who have died after they had diarrhoea?

Two

How will we collect the information?
- By asking other children in the school.
- By asking family members/members of the household.
- By asking neighbours.
- By asking a village health worker or traditional healer.

Three

How will we make a record of the information?
- Make a chart showing the names of children, their ages, the months of the year and the number of cases of diarrhoea.

Four

What can we learn from the information?
- The frequency of diarrhoea in the community.
- Which age group has diarrhoea most often.
- In which season it is most common.

Five

How can we act on the information?
- Find out more about it.
- Tell others.
- Learn how to help when children have diarrhoea.

3. An experiment ... explaining dehydration

This simple experiment demonstrates what is happening to babies' body fluids when they have diarrhoea.

Ask children to bring a small, hollow gourd to school. (If no gourd is available, an old ball, plastic bottle or anything similar will do.) Draw a mouth and some eyes on the gourd (*see illustration*). Make a hole in the top of the gourd and two small holes near the bottom, as in the drawing, to show where urine and stools come out.

- Pour in water that has some salt in it. First, pour in some water and let it all run right through. Next, keep on pouring in enough water to keep some in the gourd even while water is still running out.

- Tell children the gourd represents the body of a child who has diarrhoea. If the water in the gourd 'baby' falls too low, this causes dehydration and can cause death.

- Explain that children with diarrhoea need liquid *(see page 102 for amount)* each time they pass a loose stool, to replace the water and salt they have lost.

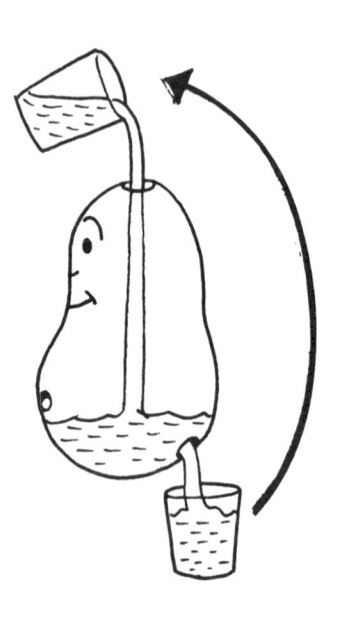

Discuss the experiment with children, using questions like:

- What happened to the water which was in the gourd baby's body?

- How can we replace the water and salt in the body that was lost through the diarrhoea?

- How do we keep enough water and salt in the body all the time? (Water and salt must be replaced every time they are lost!)

- What happens to the gourd baby's urine (from the front hole) when the water level falls below the hole?

- What happens to people, animals and plants if they have nothing to drink?

Summarize the main ideas children have learnt about dehydration, e.g.:

- When we have diarrhoea, our bodies lose a lot of water (especially if we are vomiting and have fever).
- When we lose water from our bodies, we lose salt too.
- Water and salt are essential to our bodies – if we lose too much of them and they are not replaced quickly, we will die.

4. A labelling game to help children remember the signs of severe dehydration

Children write labels describing the following signs of severe dehydration:

Sunken fontanelle.

Eyes and hands not moving.

Dry mouth and tongue.

Sunken eyes, no tears.

Loose skin.

Draw the outline of a baby on paper; on the blackboard; or on the ground.

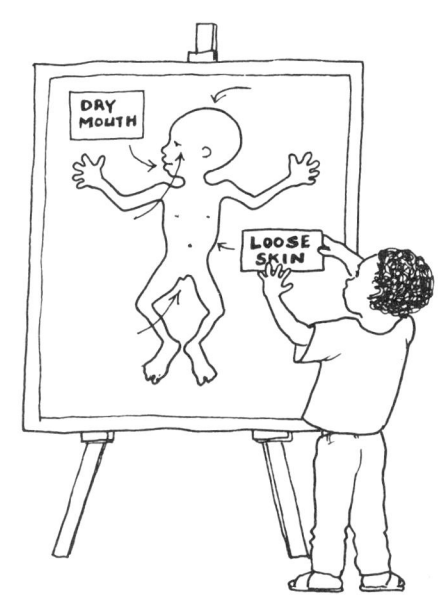

Can children think of ways to play the game: label the baby?

Remember: All games should emphasize that severely dehydrated babies need attention from a trained health worker.

5. Dramatization ... caring for children with diarrhoea

Before writing and acting the play

Discuss with children to make sure they understand the following key messages:

- It is important to be sure that children with diarrhoea drink as much liquid as they lose.
- The extra drinks should be given right from the time the diarrhoea starts.
- Giving lots of liquid to a child with diarrhoea may at first increase the amount of diarrhoea. This is natural. Most of the liquid will be absorbed and the body is trying to get rid of the germs with the diarrhoea.
- Children with diarrhoea need a drink each time they pass a loose stool (*see page 102 for amounts*).
- Getting a child to drink is not easy. We need to try, and try again, encouraging the child and giving a little of the drink at a time.

A play: *When Baby had Diarrhoea*

Ask children to make up their own play built around this outline:

- Mother and father are away.
- The older children are left to look after younger ones.
- One of them recognizes that the baby has diarrhoea.
- The nearest clinic is five miles away.
- A neighbour tells them that the baby needs an injection, but fortunately they have learnt about diarrhoea at school so they know this is wrong.
- They go to their aunt who is very sensible and who learns a lot about health at a women's group.
- She tells them the same thing that they've learnt at school ... that the baby needs lots to drink and also food.
- She comes to their home and they make the drink together (*see pages 101-102 for suggestions of suitable drinks*).
- They go on giving the baby the drink: even after it has vomited, they wait for a few minutes and then carry on giving it small sips on a spoon.
- They keep on and on, even though they are tired and it is not easy for them.
- After their parents return they go on helping to give the baby drinks and food.

☐ The baby starts to get better during the first day, but the diarrhoea continues for two more days and the children go on giving the baby extra drinks as well as food.

Don't write the words for the play. Let the children make them up but make sure they get the facts right. Talk about the different kinds of drinks that are suitable. Let them practise the play and then perform it for others.

After the play

Question children who made up the play and also those who watched it, to make sure they have remembered the key messages.

CHILDREN'S ACTION

I Can

- Help to keep food covered.
- Help to keep flies away.
- Wash my hands before eating food.
- Wash my hands after going to the latrine.
- Help other children at home to do all these things.
- Recognize when the baby has diarrhoea and tell my parents.
- Recognize danger signs (*see page 109*) and seek help from the health worker immediately.
- Explain to my family why sick babies and children need plenty of drinks, and need food as well.
- Help to prepare and give drinks, especially to babies with diarrhoea.

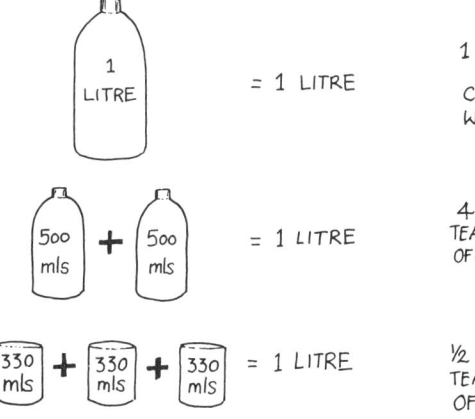

STEP 1. FIND WAYS OF MEASURING 1 LITRE (USE LOCAL CONTAINERS)

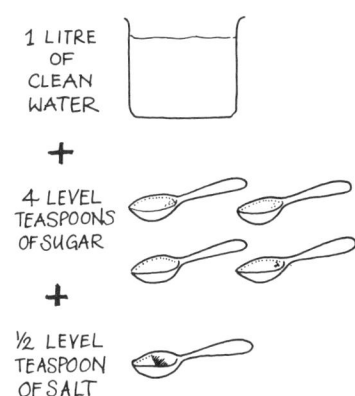

1 LITRE = 1 LITRE

500 mls + 500 mls = 1 LITRE

330 mls + 330 mls + 330 mls = 1 LITRE

STEP 2. PREPARE THE SPECIAL DRINK

1 LITRE OF CLEAN WATER

+

4 LEVEL TEASPOONS OF SUGAR

+

½ LEVEL TEASPOON OF SALT

We Can

- Organize a 'kill the fly' campaign.
- Demonstrate making a sugar and salt drink. = not described in text p102
- Perform a play at the health centre about diarrhoea.
- Demonstrate about dehydration with the gourd baby.

BASKET OF IDEAS

- Children carry out a survey, and discuss: how is diarrhoea treated – how was it treated when their grandparents were children?

- Children make a diarrhoea song and dance, and perform it. Remember, children can mime and dance insects (e.g. flies) and objects (e.g. plates of food; food covers) as well as people.

- Children find out prices and availability of recommended drinks – compare prices with those of medicines which say they help diarrhoea (but do not).

- Children take part in a poster competition based on slogans, e.g. *'Save a baby's life'*; *'Did you make baby ill?'*

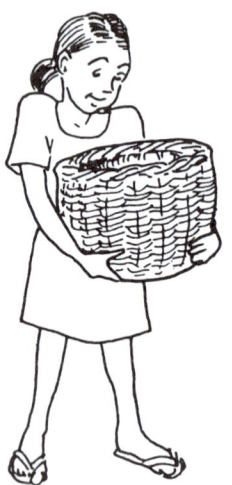

EVALUATION QUESTIONS

Children

Can we:

- Say why diarrhoea is particularly dangerous to babies?
- Recognize signs of severe dehydration?
- Say how we would help, or have already helped, to take care of a baby with diarrhoea?
- Make a rehydration drink?
- Recognize the taste of the right solution?
- Say what rehydration drinks are available and can be used in our families?
- Describe what we are doing to prevent diarrhoea through better hygiene?

Teachers
- Do children know what rehydration drinks are available, and how to make them?
- Have children demonstrated what they have learnt at home? How did parents react?
- Has the school taken action to prevent children getting diarrhoea (e.g. cleaner latrines, fewer flies)?

Health Workers
- Have children spread messages to the community (e.g. plays, songs, campaigns)?
- Have any effects been observed which might have been a result of children's knowledge and action (e.g. fewer deaths of babies; more severe cases brought to the clinic)?

What children need to know and pass on about
Immunization

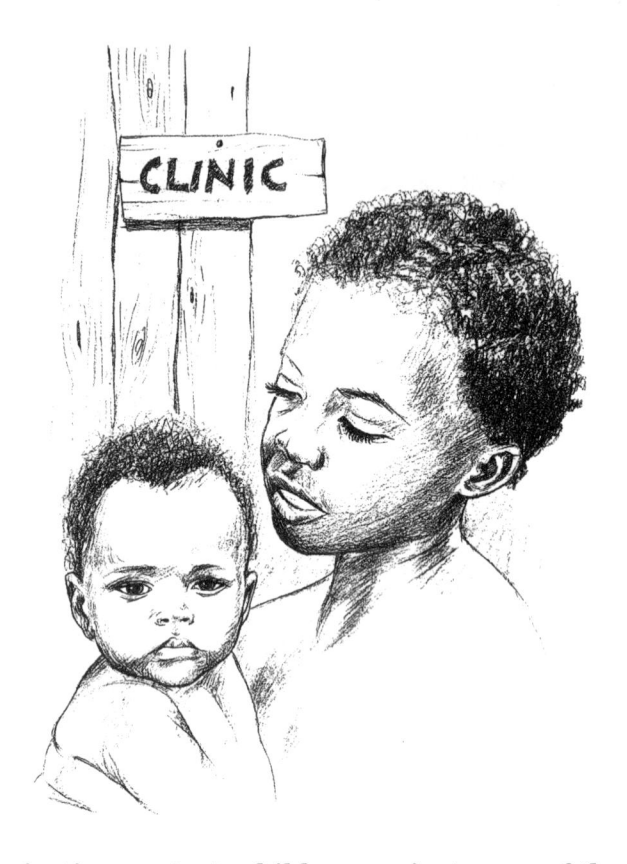

Immunization protects children against some of the most dangerous diseases of childhood. Without immunization, many children die or become disabled.

Immunization campaigns worldwide have already helped to save millions of lives and children in many countries have played a part in them. However, much more needs to be done to persuade all families to bring all children to be immunized at the right time, and to complete the full course of immunizations.

Children are among the most powerful agents to communicate these messages and help their parents to make full use of immunization services.

PRIME MESSAGES
and supporting information

1 | Immunization protects against several dangerous diseases. A child who is not immunized is more likely to become undernourished, to become disabled, and to die.

● Immunization protects children against some of the most dangerous diseases of childhood. A child is immunized by vaccines which are injected or given by mouth. The vaccines work by building up the child's defences. If the disease strikes before a child is immunized, immunization is too late.

● A child who is not immunized is very likely to get measles and whooping cough. These diseases can kill. But even children who survive these diseases are weakened by them. They may not grow well. And they may die later from malnutrition or other illnesses.

● Measles is also an important cause of malnutrition, poor mental growth, and blindness.

● An unimmunized child will almost certainly be infected with the polio virus. And for every 200 children who are infected, one will be crippled for life.

● Tetanus germs grow in dirty cuts and kill most of the people who become infected – if they are not immunized.

● Breastfeeding is a kind of natural immunization against several diseases. Some of the mother's resistance to disease is passed to the child in her breastmilk, and especially in the thick yellow milk (called colostrum) which is produced during the first few days after the birth.

2 | Immunization is urgent. All immunizations should be completed in the first year of the child's life.

● It is vital to immunize children early in life. Half of all deaths from whooping cough, one third of all cases of polio, and a quarter of all deaths from measles, occur before the age of one year.

● It is vital for infants to complete the full course of immunizations, otherwise the vaccines may not work. Some vaccines need to be given only once. Others have to be given three times, with a gap of at least four weeks between each dose.

● The important thing for parents to know is that a child should be taken for immunization five times in the first year of the child's life:

- At birth, or as soon as possible afterwards, babies should be immunized against tuberculosis.
- In countries where polio is still a problem, newborn babies can also be given a dose of polio vaccine. This is in addition to the three doses given at the ages of six, 10 and 14 weeks.
- At the age of six weeks, parents should bring their babies for a first immunization against diphtheria, whooping cough, and tetanus. These three vaccines are given together in a single injection called DPT. The first of three doses of polio vaccine should also be given at this time.
- At the ages of 10 and 14 weeks, parents should return for their infants to complete the full course of DPT and polio vaccines.
- As soon as possible after the age of nine months, parents should bring their babies for immunization against measles.

● Measles is one of the most dangerous of all childhood diseases. For the first few months of life, the child has some natural protection against measles. This natural protection is inherited from the child's mother. It may prevent measles vaccination from doing its job. But after about nine months, natural protection comes to an end. The child is now at risk from measles and can and should be immunized. So it is vital to take a child for measles vaccination as soon as possible after the age of nine months.

● If for any reason a child has not been fully immunized in the first year of life, it is vital to have the child immunized as soon as possible.

	Immunization schedule for infants*
AGE	DISEASE TO BE IMMUNIZED AGAINST
Birth	Tuberculosis (and polio in some countries)
6 weeks	Diphtheria, whooping cough, tetanus, polio
10 weeks	Diphtheria, whooping cough, tetanus, polio
14 weeks	Diphtheria, whooping cough, tetanus, polio
9 months	Measles (12-15 months in industrialized countries) and polio in some countries
	* National immunization schedules may differ slightly from country to country.

3 | It is safe to immunize a sick child.

● One of the main reasons why parents do not bring their children for immunization is that the child has a fever, a cough, a cold, diarrhoea, or some other mild illness on the day the child is to be immunized. Even if the child with a case of mild illness or malnutrition is brought for immunization, health workers may advise against giving the injections. This is wrong advice. It is now known that it is safe to immunize a child who is suffering from a minor illness or malnutrition.

● After an injection the child may cry, develop a fever, a rash, or a small sore. As with any illness, a child should be given plenty of food and liquids. Breastfeeding is especially helpful. If the problem seems serious or lasts more than three days, the child should be taken to a health centre.

4 | Every woman between the ages of 15 and 44 should be fully immunized against tetanus.

● In many parts of the world, mothers give birth in unhygienic conditions. This puts both mother and child at risk from tetanus, a major killer of the newborn. If the mother is not immunized against tetanus, then one baby in every 100 will die from the disease.

● Tetanus germs grow in dirty cuts. This can happen, for example, if an unclean knife is used to cut the umbilical cord or if anything unclean is put on the stump of the cord. (Anything used to cut the cord should first be cleaned and then boiled or heated in a flame and allowed to cool.)

If the tetanus germs enter the mother's body, and if she is not immunized against tetanus, then her life will also be at risk.

● All women of child-bearing age should be immunized against tetanus. All women who become pregnant should check to make sure they have been immunized against tetanus. In this way, both mothers and their newborn babies will be protected.

● If a woman is not already immunized, a first dose of tetanus vaccine should be given as soon as she becomes pregnant. The second dose can be given four weeks after the first. This second dose should be given *before* the last two weeks of the pregnancy.

A third dose should be given six to 12 months after the second dose, or during the next pregnancy.

These three tetanus vaccinations protect the mother, and her newborn baby, for five years. All infants should be immunized against tetanus during the first year of life.

● If a girl or a woman has been vaccinated five times against tetanus, then she is protected against the disease throughout her years of child-bearing. Any children she may then have will also be protected for the first few weeks of life.

OBJECTIVES for children's understanding and action

Children should:

● Understand that all children need to be protected by immunization against six killer diseases (tuberculosis, diphtheria, whooping cough, tetanus, polio, measles); and that immunization should be completed in the first year of a child's life.

● Understand the dangers of not immunizing children.

● Know the national immunization schedule; and when and where immunization takes place locally.

● Know how to spread the immunization message; and help their families when they take children to the clinic.

UNDERSTANDING about immunization

1. Story-telling ... what happened to children who were not immunized?

Tell stories to help children understand that:

☐ Babies must be immunized against the six killer diseases.

☐ Babies should be immunized in their first year of life.

☐ Babies who are not immunized against these diseases may get very sick and die.

Make up a story or build one from these outlines:

☐ *Our village is not far from the health centre. The immunization clinic takes place regularly. Most families bring their children, but one family never goes. They are among the most successful farmers in the community. The father is strong and healthy.*

'Why should I take my children to the clinic?' he laughs. 'The clinic is for sick people. We are happy and lucky. Our children will not be ill.'

They had a daughter aged 10 who went to school. When the youngest baby was born, she pleaded with her parents to take him to the clinic as she had learned about immunization, but they would not listen to her. Then there was an epidemic of polio in the village. The baby and an older boy of three became sick. Neither died but both are severely disabled. The baby may never be able to walk.

- *I live in a town with my mother, brother and baby sister. Our father went away. We do not see him any more. The baby is still small and when she was six weeks old my mother took her to be immunized. She was told to come back four weeks later for the baby's second immunization. But when the time came my baby sister had a cold and our neighbour advised my mother not to take her to the clinic. My mother never took my sister to the clinic after that. I think she was worried about what the health worker would say to her.*

  Then our neighbour's boy caught whooping cough, and our baby caught it too. She has been coughing, vomiting, losing weight and becoming weak. Sometimes she goes blue with the cough. The health worker has told my mother that our baby may die.

- *We live in a big house outside town. My family is rich and there were only two of us, me and my brother who was one year old. I know my parents took him to be immunized four times when he was very small, but I don't think they ever took him for a measles immunization when he was nine months. He was so healthy and I heard my uncle tell them that healthy children don't need to be taken.*

  Then last month I caught measles. I wasn't very sick, but then my brother caught it. It was terrible. He had a high fever for six days with red eyes, a runny nose, noisy breathing and a cough. He had a rash all over. On the sixth day his breathing got worse. They told me he had caught pneumonia. Two doctors came to the house. They tried to save him. It was too late, and now my baby brother is dead.

Remember that whichever story you use, it will work better if:

- You make sure the children understand the language.
- The story has some excitement, action and drama in it.
- The story shows children what they themselves can achieve as a group.
- It captures their interest because it appeals to their sense of

adventure, or their desire to help, or is about something important to them.

Involve the children in the story right from the beginning and help them to contribute to it. Here are some suggestions:

- The children can name the characters and the story itself.
- Give them something to look for in the story before you begin: 'I want you to tell me why the child was not immunized.'
- Allow them to predict the action: 'Well, she can do three things, what do you think she will do?'
- Invite their suggestions: 'Who would listen to him? What do you think they should do?'
- When the story is over, ask them to consider alternatives: 'Suppose she had immunized the baby, what might have happened?' 'Would the story be different if people in the community knew all the facts about immunization?'
- You need to make sure that they have understood the health message. To help them remember the messages in the story you can do some of these things:

  Help the children to draw the story in a series of pictures which they can mix up and put back in the right order.

  Help them to make their own story book complete with pictures and cover.

  Ask a group of children to tell the story, each contributing a part, or to tell the story from different characters' points of view.

2. Role-play ... why have children not been immunized?

Children discuss in class and list the reasons why families do not immunize their children and why the reasons are wrong.

Then they form groups and pretend to be adults. One gives a reason for not immunizing their child. The others try to convince them to do so.

3. Finding out ... who has been immunized in our families?

Which children in class have brothers and sisters under two years old? Have they all been immunized? (Children check with their families and report back.)

If babies have not been immunized, what was the reason? What action can be taken?

4. Finding out ... about immunization programmes in the community

Against which diseases does the immunization programme protect children? (Find posters or leaflets.)

At what ages does the programme recommend that immunization should be given?

Where and when are immunizations given? How do people find out about them?

CHILDREN'S ACTION

I Can

● Make a birthday card to take home for a new baby in the family or neighbourhood, and hang on the wall as a reminder. The class can help to design the card, so that it shows the right times for the local immunization programme.

YOUR IMMUNISATION CARD	
HAPPY BIRTHDAY (WRITE THE BABY'S NAME HERE)	TICK OR COLOUR THE SPACE FOR EACH IMMUNIZATION GIVEN
WE HOPE YOU HAVE ALREADY HAD YOUR FIRST **POLIO, & TB VACCINE**	
AT SIX WEEKS OLD YOU NEED **DPT & POLIO**	
AT 2½ MONTHS OLD YOU NEED **DPT & POLIO**	
AT 3 - 4 MONTHS OLD YOU NEED **DPT & POLIO**	
BEFORE YOU ARE 1 YEAR OLD YOU NEED **MEASLES**	

● Keep reminding mother and father to look at the baby's clinic card and the birthday card, to remind them when immunizations are due.

● Help to take the baby to the clinic for immunization, at the right time.

● After the immunization, help to look after babies and comfort them if they feel unwell and cry.

● Look after other children when mother goes to the clinic.

We Can

● Make posters about immunization and display them in a place where everyone will see them.

● Make up and perform plays about what happens when someone in the family is not immunized and gets one of the diseases which can be prevented. (The play might show the unpleasant and crafty germs who wait around for those who have not been immunized. They include Measles Germ [with red spots], Polio Germ [who limps], Whooping Cough Germ and TB Germ [who cough]. Some children can take the parts of the germs; others can be the antibodies.)

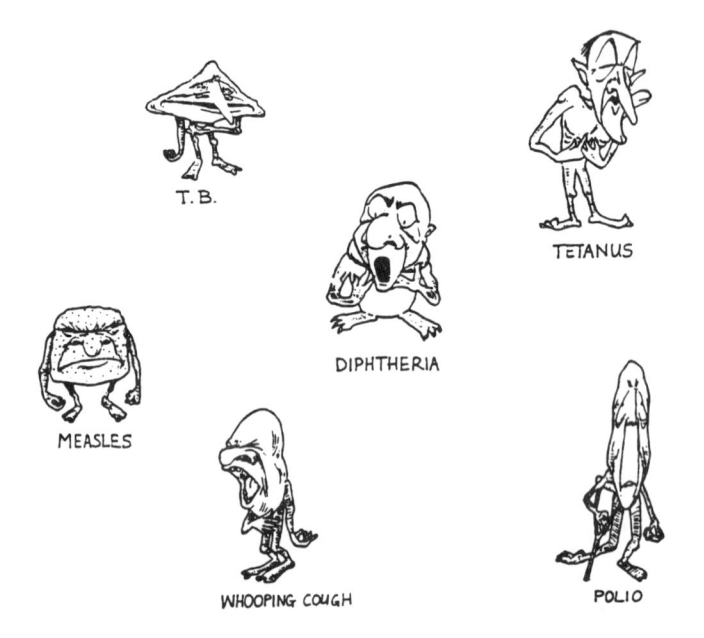

T.B.

TETANUS

DIPHTHERIA

MEASLES

WHOOPING COUGH

POLIO

● With our teachers, support the clinic by keeping records for all the families of the children in the class, or if possible for all the families in the village.

● Help others to know about immunization programmes and prepare, with adults, for the visit of the immunization team or health worker to the community.

● Take responsibility for a group of families nearby to ensure that they understand about immunization and bring all their children to be immunized. Go on a march carrying a placard to announce the immunization times.

BASKET OF IDEAS

● Children ask their grandparents what happened before immunization.

● Children count how many people are disabled by polio – in their age group, and among people who are 10 and 20 years older. Is there any difference? Why?

● Children help others who are disabled.

● Children take part in a story-telling competition with immunization messages. They present the best stories at an open day or a local festival.

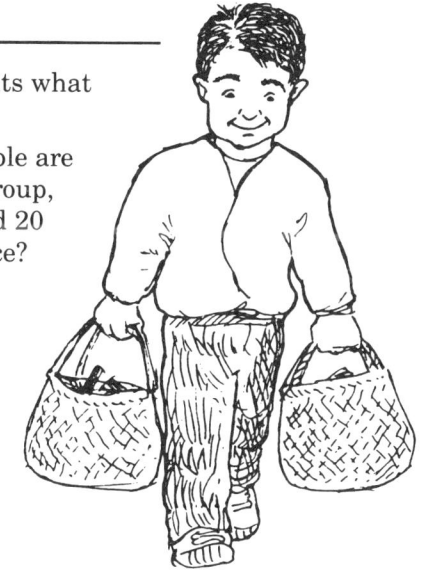

EVALUATION QUESTIONS

Children

- Do we all remember and understand the immunization message?
- Do I know the times at the clinic for immunization?
- Have children at home under two years old been properly immunized?

Teachers

- Can children list the six killer diseases, and when babies should be immunized against them?
- Have children continued to make record cards for new babies?
- Are the cards kept up to date?
- Have children made and displayed posters, and made up and performed plays about immunization?

Health Workers

- Have we involved children in immunization campaigns?
- Do we have plans to involve them regularly?

What children need to know and pass on about
Coughs and Colds

Demonstrating breathing rates with a simple pendulum

Everyone gets coughs and colds. Most coughs and colds get better without special medicine. But sometimes colds turn to pneumonia. Four million children die of pneumonia every year.

The clearest sign of pneumonia that everyone can learn to recognize is QUICK BREATHING. Pneumonia needs immediate treatment with special medicine given only by a doctor or health worker.

Breastfeeding, good food, a smoke-free home, and immunization against whooping cough, measles and diphtheria can help prevent pneumonia.

Children can help others with coughs and colds recover and grow strong by making sure they have good food and plenty to drink. They can also learn to recognize the danger signs of pneumonia so that babies at risk can get medical help quickly.

PRIME MESSAGES
and supporting information

1 If a child with a cough is breathing much more rapidly than normal, then the child is at risk. It is essential to get the child to a clinic quickly.

● Most coughs and colds, sore throats and runny noses will get better by themselves. But sometimes pneumonia develops and threatens the child's life. Millions of child deaths from pneumonia could be avoided if:

　□ Parents know when a cough or cold is becoming a serious infection that needs medical attention.

　□ Medical help and low-cost drugs are available.

● Parents of a child with a cough should know that it is essential to get the child to a clinic or a trained health worker quickly if:

　□ The child is breathing much more rapidly than normal (over 50 times a minute).

　□ The lower part of the child's chest (the area between the two halves of the child's ribcage) goes in as the child breathes in instead of expanding outwards as normal.

☐ The child is unable to drink anything.

● If a child is breathing normally, coughs and colds and runny noses can be treated at home without drugs. Most medicines sold for coughs and colds are useless or harmful.

2 | **Families can help prevent pneumonia by making sure that babies are breastfed for at least the first six months of life and that all children are well nourished and fully immunized.**

● **Breastfeeding**

Breastmilk helps to protect against infections. On average, babies who are bottle-fed have twice as many bouts of pneumonia as babies who are breastfed. It is particularly important to give breastmilk alone for about the first six months of a baby's life.

● **Feeding**

At any age, a child who is well fed is less likely to become seriously ill or to die because of pneumonia.

● **Vitamin A**

Vitamin A, from orange or yellow fruits and dark green leafy vegetables, also helps to protect against pneumonia.

● **Immunization**

Immunization should be completed before the child is one year old. The child will then be protected against some of the most common causes of serious respiratory infections, including whooping cough, tuberculosis and measles.

● **Crowding**

Overcrowding helps the spread of coughs and colds. At night, infants who are breastfed can sleep with the mother. But older children should be encouraged to sleep on their own.

3 | **A child with a cough or cold should be helped to eat and to drink plenty of liquids.**

Important things to remember when treating a child at home are to:

● **Continue feeding**

A breastfed child with a cough or cold may be difficult to feed. But feeding helps both to fight the infection and to protect the child's growth. So it is important to persist in frequent attempts to give breastmilk. Clearing the child's blocked nose will help the child to suck. If a child cannot suck, it is best to squeeze out the breastmilk and feed the child from a clean cup.

Children who are not being breastfed should be coaxed into eating frequent small amounts. Periods of 'starvation' caused by illness and lost appetite are a major reason for poor growth. When the illness is over, a child should be fed an extra meal each day for a week. Recovery is not complete until the child is at least the same weight as when the illness began.

● Give plenty of fluids

All children with coughs and colds need to drink plenty of liquids.

4 | A child with a cough or cold should be kept warm but not hot, and should breathe clean, non-smoky air.

● Keep warm not hot

Babies and very young children lose their heat easily, so it is important to keep them covered and warm, but not too hot or too tightly wrapped.

Fever is not always a sign of severe illness. But if a child has a fever, paracetamol (or other temperature-reducing medicine) can be given.

● Help in breathing

A child's nose should be frequently cleared, especially before breastfeeding or when being put to sleep. A moist atmosphere can help to ease breathing. It can also help if the child inhales water vapour from a bowl of hot but not boiling water.

The air in the child's room should be kept fresh by opening a door or window two or three times a day. But a child with a cough or cold should be kept away from draughts.

● Clean air

Children who live and sleep in smoky surroundings, either because of cooking fires or tobacco smoking, are more likely to get pneumonia. Tobacco smoke in the air that a child breathes can cause long-term damage to the child's health.

Spitting and sneezing by other people close to children also increases the risk. People with coughs and colds should be kept away from young babies.

OBJECTIVES for children's understanding and action

Children should:

● Understand that most coughs and colds get better on their own and that most medicines sold for coughs and colds are useless or harmful.

● Know how to help children with coughs and colds by giving them good food and plenty of drinks, and keeping them warm and away from smoky places.

● Be able to recognize the danger signs of pneumonia in babies and young children, and know that they should be taken to a health worker immediately.

● Know that children are less likely to get pneumonia if they are breastfed, well nourished, protected by adequate vitamin A, and immunized against whooping cough, measles and diphtheria.

UNDERSTANDING about coughs, colds and pneumonia

1. A story or play, followed by discussion and drawing ... right and wrong ways of treating a cold

Present the following outline:

The Market 'Doctor'

☐ A child gets a heavy cold and makes a big fuss.

☐ His family take him to the market.

☐ A 'doctor' is there with his own medicines including a strong and very expensive antibiotic. Injections cost even more, and he always recommends them.

☐ The family choose an injection.

☐ The child's arm swells up and the cold gets no better.

☐ They consult the health worker who tells them they have wasted their money and put their child at risk. She recommends the right practices (*refer back to objectives and Facts for Life messages*) and advises the family to buy and grow more fruit and green vegetables to help protect children against coughs and colds in future.

Children make either plays or stories, based on the outline.

They discuss the play or story in relation to their own experience, and draw a series of pictures to illustrate it.

2. A discussion about pneumonia led by the health worker

Invite the health worker to come to the school and talk to the children about pneumonia.

Follow the talk by a discussion reinforcing children's knowledge and relating it to their own experience. The following questions may be included:

- How can we tell the difference between a bad cold and pneumonia?
- What are the signs and symptoms of pneumonia?
- Do we know anyone who has had pneumonia? For how long? What time of the year was it? Did it start on its own, or follow from a cold, or from measles, diphtheria or whooping cough? Did it get better? What helped? Was any medicine made at home, or did it come from the doctor or health worker?

From the discussion children should learn that:

- All children (and also adults) can get pneumonia, but babies under one year are more likely to get it than older children.
- Pneumonia can start on its own, follow from a cold, or follow from measles, diphtheria or whooping cough.
- The clearest and surest sign of pneumonia is quick breathing. A healthy baby, lying still and not crying, takes about 30 breaths a minute. But a baby with pneumonia, lying quietly, takes more than 50 breaths a minute, and persistently breathes at this rate (for over 10 minutes).
- Other signs are also important and easy to recognize (*see pages 125-126*).

3. How to count breaths

We need to learn how to count breaths to be sure to recognize quick breathing. (Mothers usually know when their babies are breathing too fast even without a watch.)

• **Counting breaths**

If a watch or clock is available, children work in pairs, counting each other's breaths for one minute. They write down the number of breaths. Then one child does any activity from List A, the other any activity from List B. They count each other's breaths after each activity, then change over and continue, each time writing down the result.

A	B
Sitting quietly	Running on the spot very fast
Reading	Skipping 30 times
Standing still	Jumping as high as possible 30 times
Humming	Stepping on and off a chair or bench 30 times
Writing	Lifting something heavy
Digging	Counting

By comparing different rates of breathing, children soon begin to understand what is normal and what is fast breathing.

If they do not have a watch or clock, a third child can act as timekeeper, counting up to 100 at a steady speed, or walking up and down at the same pace. Children can compare the rate of breathing for different activities, even if they cannot measure accurately.

- **Making pendulums**

Children make pendulums from string which does not stretch, and stones. The string should be 225cm long before the stone is tied on. Then three loops should be tied: 35 cm from the stone; one metre from the stone; and two metres from the stone.

Children hold the loop and swing the pendulum. The stone swings from side to side. All the children should breathe in time with the stone: breathe in as it swings one way; and breathe out as it swings the other way:

> 21 times per minute when the string is two metres long (a normal adult's, or older child's, rate of breathing).

> 30 times per minute when the string is one metre long (a normal baby's rate of breathing).

> 50 times per minute when the string is 35 cm long. This is the rate at which a baby with pneumonia breathes. **Danger! If a baby breathes at this rate for over 10 minutes, it should be taken to a health worker fast**.

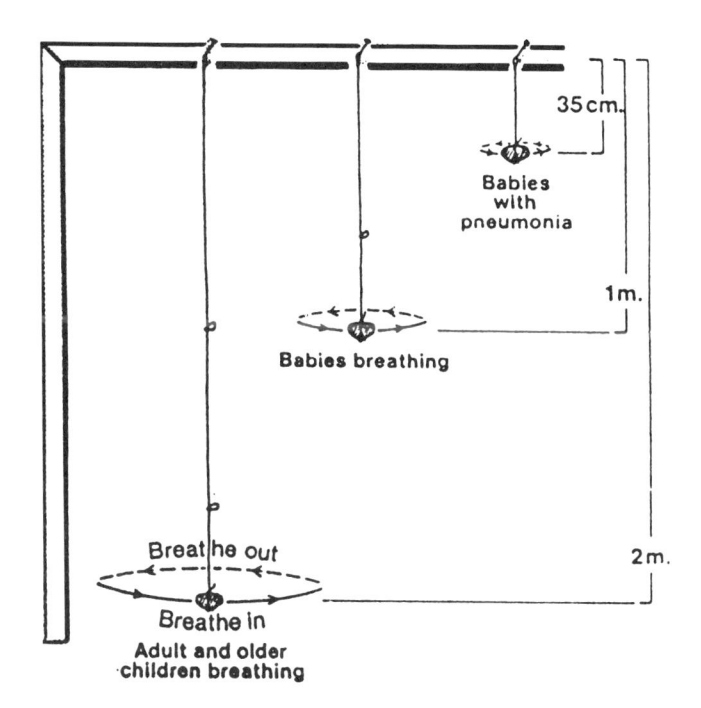

CHILDREN'S ACTION

I Can

● Encourage little brothers and sisters to eat and drink when they are feeling unwell with coughs and colds.

● Tell my family what I have learned about the signs of pneumonia.

● Count the breaths of little brothers and sisters when they are feeling very unwell and know the danger signs so that they can be taken to a health worker or doctor quickly.

We Can

● Help to grow orange and yellow fruits, and green leafy vegetables.

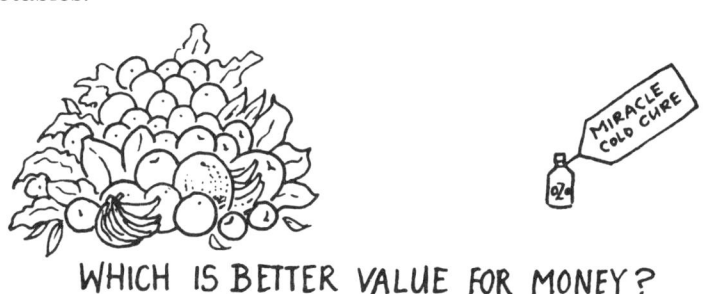

WHICH IS BETTER VALUE FOR MONEY?

- Make and display posters with messages about preventing and treating coughs and colds, e.g. *'Spitting, coughs and sneezes spread diseases'*; *'It's better to spend your money on good food than expensive medicines for coughs and colds'*.

- Make up a song/play/puppet play with messages about recognizing pneumonia. Perform it to the rest of the school and to parents.

BASKET OF IDEAS

- Teachers organize a simple survey so that children find out how many of them have a cold and a cough, or both. How many brothers, sisters, parents and grandparents have colds or coughs? Do several people in one family have a cold or a cough? How many of those that cough, smoke? Do babies or old people have more colds and coughs? Children make a chart to display the results of the survey.

- Children find out the prices of medicines sold for coughs and colds in the shops and market. How much good food can the family buy instead of a bottle of medicine?

- Children write a story about a child who notices that the baby shows signs of pneumonia. How does the child convince older people to take the baby to the health worker?

EVALUATION QUESTIONS

Children
- Can we remember how to help a child with a cough or a cold?
- Can we list which good foods help to prevent coughs and colds?
- Have we tested each other to see if we can recognize fast breathing?

Teachers
- Do most children know the danger signs when coughs and colds might be pneumonia?

- Do they know what to do and where to seek help?
- What action have children taken to pass on messages?

Health Workers

- Have we helped schools to pass on the right information?
- Have any families taken action as a result?

What children need to know and pass on about Malaria

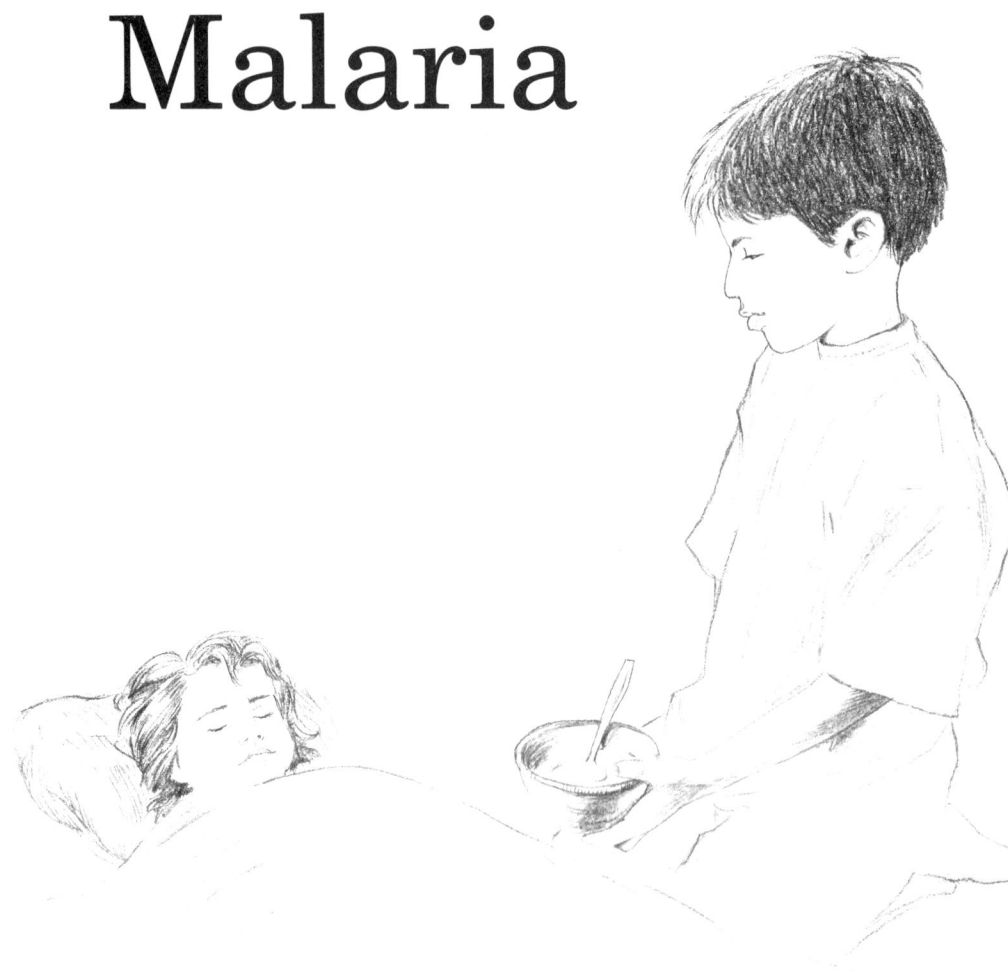

My little sister has fever

Malaria affects millions of people worldwide and kills large numbers of children. Children are particularly at risk when they are made weak by other diseases and poor nutrition.

Children can contribute to national malaria control programmes by helping to prevent mosquitoes from breeding and biting people.

They can also learn how to help a child with fever by preventing the temperature from rising too high and giving the sick child plenty of liquids.

PRIME MESSAGES and supporting information

Preventing and managing malaria

1 | **Young children should be protected from mosquito bites, especially at night.**

- Malaria is spread by the bite of a mosquito. Care should be taken to keep mosquitoes away from young children. There are several ways of doing this:
    - By using bed nets (preferably impregnated with a mosquito repellent).
    - By using fumigants such as mosquito coils.
    - By putting screens on house windows and doors.
    - By killing mosquitoes in the house.
- All members of the community should be protected against mosquito bites. A mosquito can pick up malaria from an infected person and pass it on to someone who is uninfected.

2 | **Communities should destroy mosquito larvae and prevent mosquitoes from breeding.**

- Mosquitoes breed wherever stagnant water can collect: in ponds, swamps, pools, pits, drains, sometimes even tin cans and hoof-prints. They may also breed along the edges of streams, in overhead tanks, and in rice fields. Filling in or draining places where water collects can kill the mosquito larvae. Overhead tanks can be covered. The larvae in rice fields can be killed by alternately drying out the field and introducing larvae-eating fish into the water.
- Regular clean-ups of the neighbourhood help to reduce mosquito breeding.

3 | **Wherever malaria is common, pregnant women should take anti-malarial tablets throughout pregnancy.**

- Pregnant women are more than twice as likely to suffer from malaria. The disease is also more dangerous during pregnancy. It can lead to severe anaemia ('thin blood'), and may cause a miscarriage, premature birth, or stillbirth. Babies born to women with malaria are also very likely to be small, weak, and vulnerable to infections.

● Pregnant women can be effectively protected against malaria by taking anti-malarial tablets regularly throughout pregnancy.

● Anti-malarial tablets should be obtained from a clinic or health worker as not all anti-malarials are safe to take during pregnancy.

4 | Wherever malaria is common, a child who has a fever should be taken immediately to a health worker. If malaria appears to be the cause, the child should be given a full course of an anti-malarial drug.

● A child with a fever, believed to be caused by malaria, should be given a course of anti-malarial tablets (young babies may be given an anti-malarial syrup). Treatment for malaria should begin immediately. Even a day's delay can be fatal. A health worker can advise on what type of treatment is best and how long it should last.

● A child should be given the full course of treatment, even if the fever disappears rapidly.

If the symptoms continue, the child should be taken to a health centre or hospital – the malaria may be resistant to the drugs.

Nursing children with fever (from malaria or other causes)

5 | A child with a fever must drink frequently. ORS solution replaces salt as well as water lost through sweating.

● When children have fever, they sweat. Sweating is important because it helps to cool them by evaporation. But they also lose water from their bodies.

● A child with fever needs to drink frequently and this drink needs to put back the salt which has been lost, as well as the water. ORS drinks should therefore be given to children with fever.

6 | A child with a fever should be kept cool but not cold. A child with a very high temperature (fever) is in danger of fits which can cause brain damage.

● Malaria and other infections can cause a very high temperature

136

and make a child have fits (convulsions). If the fits go on for more than 10 minutes they can lead to brain damage, particularly in young children and babies.

● When a child has a very high temperature this should be brought down immediately by:

- Giving a temperature-reducing medicine (such as paracetamol).
- Removing the child's clothes. Never put many clothes or blankets on children with fever.
- Sponging, particularly the forehead, hands and feet. If necessary, bathe the child in cool (not cold) water.

These activities will also prevent a moderate temperature going very high.

7 | **A child recovering from a fever (or other disease) needs plenty of liquids and food.**

● A fever, from malaria or other causes, burns up energy and the child loses a lot of liquid through sweating. Once children are willing to eat, they should be encouraged to eat plenty to make up for the food missed while they had a poor appetite. They should continue to drink plenty.

N.B. Some of the prime messages and supporting information in this section have been expanded in order to give more information about nursing children with fever.

OBJECTIVES for children's understanding and action

Children should:

● Understand that malaria is spread by mosquitoes which breed in stagnant water and bite at night, spreading germs from infected to healthy people.

● Know how to prevent malaria by stopping mosquitoes breeding and biting; and understand that bed nets impregnated with a mosquito repellent are the best means of protection against mosquito bites.

● Understand that malaria can be treated by anti-malarial tablets available from a health worker and that the full course of tablets must be taken.

- Know how to help a child with a fever by keeping them cool but not cold.
- Understand that children with a fever need plenty of drinks to replace the water and salt they have lost through sweating.
- Know how to help a child recover by giving plenty of liquids and extra food for at least a week afterwards.

UNDERSTANDING about malaria and fever

1. Making a map* of places around the school or the neighbourhood where mosquitoes might breed

From this children can learn to:
- Identify places where mosquitoes are likely to breed.
- Check the places where water collects to see if they have larvae.
- Plan actions to destroy potential breeding places.

Before making the map, ask the children to:
- List the kinds of places where they might find mosquito larvae.
- Decide how they will record what they find.
- Decide how they will work as a group to investigate and to record.
- Discuss and decide who they need to ask for permission and how they can ask with courtesy.

Organize the investigation
- Decide the best time for the investigation.
- Set a time limit on it.
- Supervise children's safety especially if the investigation is outside the school compound.

Help children make the map
- Children use their findings and make a map to show the places they have found where mosqito larvae might breed.
- They display their maps and discuss their findings, e.g. Where are the spots that are potential breeding places? Where did we find mosquito larvae? What actions can we take to prevent mosquitoes breeding in these places?

---

*There are many ways to make a map – it can be drawn on the ground, on the blackboard, on large pieces of paper for display, on graph paper or in the children's books; it can be modelled with clay or scrap material.

2. A survey ... how do we treat children who have fever?
Plan which questions to ask

Children may need to ask some of the following:
- How do families decide whether a child has fever?
- How do they decide when to take the child to the health worker?
- How do families treat and nurse a child with fever? (Ask about medicines and drinks given; and whether children are kept cool, or covered with blankets.)
- Are children fed during and after fever? If so, how?

Decide how to record the information
- Make a questionnaire with enough space to record answers.

After the survey is completed
- Discuss the results.
- Discuss and decide what information children can pass on, and to whom, about what they have learnt.

3. Drawing or miming the malaria cycle
Explain the four steps in the malaria cycle:
- Mosquito bites person with malaria (at night).
- Healthy mosquito sucks in parasites.
- Malaria parasite develops inside mosquito.
- Healthy person is bitten by malarial mosquito and gets malaria.

Children in groups decide how to present this information to each other. They can draw it, mime it, or sing it.

CHILDREN'S ACTION

I Can
- Kill mosquitoes in the house.
- Make sure that nets are properly used.
- Make sure that younger children stay under the nets until first light and that nets are well tucked in.
- Check regularly for holes and tears in nets and sew them up (but even nets with some holes help to prevent malaria particularly if they have been impregnated).

● When the spray teams come, help carry food and other things out of the house.

● Care for children with fever ... wipe them with a cloth to cool them, give plenty of drinks or the ORS drink, and food to make them strong. When the health worker has prescribed medicine, help make sure that children take the full course.

We Can

● Destroy mosquito larvae. Fill in or drain places where mosquitoes breed.

● Make and fit covers for water pots and containers.

● Act, mime or dance, at a school open day:
- The life cycle of a mosquito.
- Careless and careful families and villages (some can act the part of clever mosquitoes).
- How to care for a child with fever.

● Make posters to show:
- How malaria is spread.
- How it can be controlled.
- That children need to take the full course of medicine.

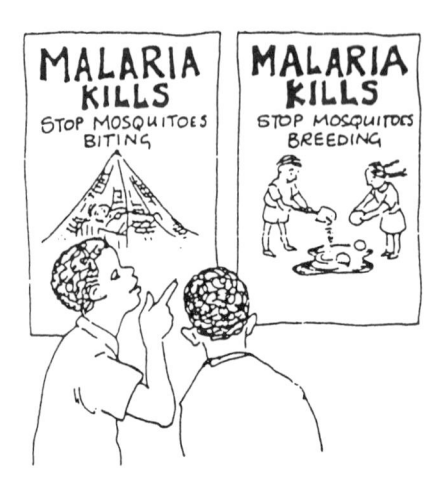

BASKET OF IDEAS

● In mathematics, children make graphs of the increase and decline of malaria in different seasons of a year, either in one school or based on records from the health centre.

● In social studies, children do surveys and make maps (where are there most cases of malaria? where do mosquitoes breed?)

● In science, children learn about the life cycle of the mosquito.

● In language, children write stories and plays about malaria, and share them with others. Some titles might be:

　□ *Mrs Mosquito and Her Friends.*
　□ *The Day the Spray Team Came to Our Village.*
　□ *Careless Moses* (who did not take the full course of medicine).

● In cultural subjects, children make up songs and dances, and draw pictures.

● The agricultural worker tells the children about breeding fish which destroy mosquito larvae.

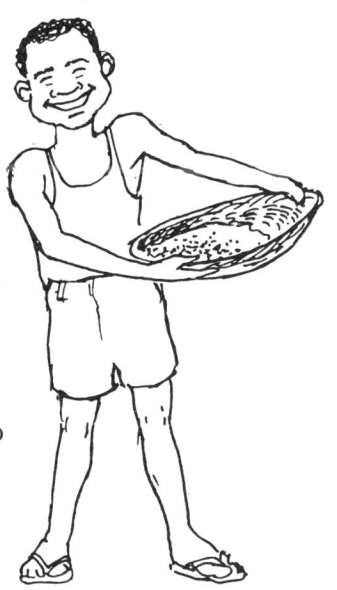

EVALUATION QUESTIONS

Children

- Do we know how malaria is spread and how it can be prevented?
- Have we taken any action to prevent mosquitoes breeding and biting?
- Do we know how to look after a child with fever?

Teachers

- Do children know which mosquitoes carry malaria, when they bite, and how the malaria germ is passed from one person to another?
- Have we included messages about malaria in different subjects across the curriculum?

Health Workers

- Have children helped to spread new knowledge about how to nurse children with fever (e.g. keep children cool not hot; give drinks and food)?

What children need to know and pass on about
AIDS

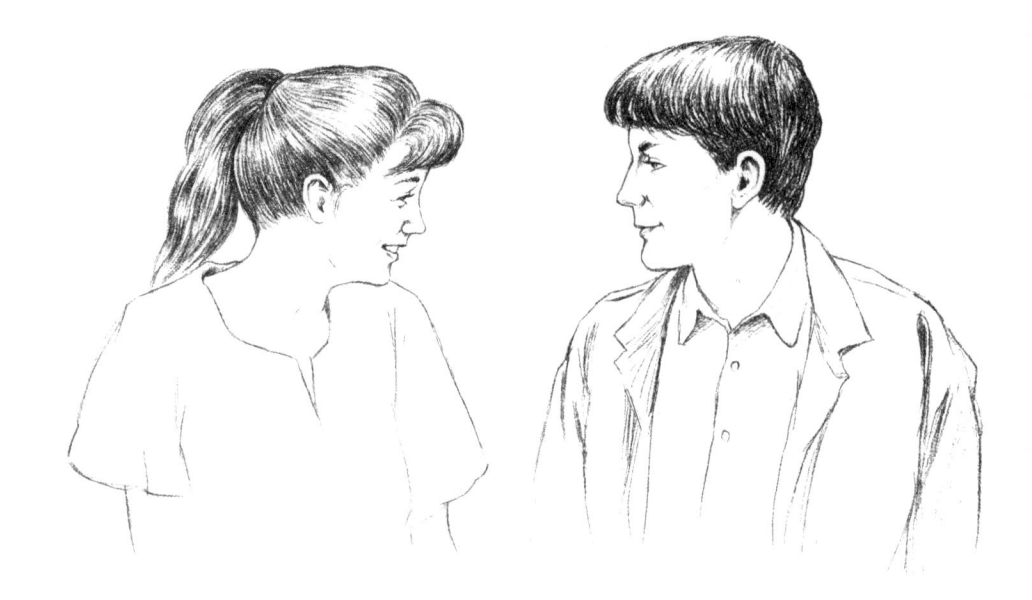

How can we stay safe?

AIDS is at present incurable. HIV, the virus which causes AIDS, kills by damaging the body's defences against other diseases.

Millions of people worldwide are infected, and numbers are rising every year. Increasing numbers of babies are being born with HIV. In addition, millions of uninfected children will be orphaned by AIDS during the 1990s.

At the moment, the only effective weapon against the spread of AIDS is public education. That is why every person in every country should know how to avoid getting and spreading HIV.

Children have a key role in protecting themselves, spreading messages to others, and helping those who have AIDS or who have been left without parents. In order to do this, they must understand how the virus which causes AIDS is acquired and spread.

PRIME MESSAGES
and supporting information

1 | AIDS is an incurable disease. It is caused by a virus which can be passed on by sexual intercourse, by infected blood, and by infected mothers to their unborn children.

- AIDS is caused by a virus known as the human immunodeficiency virus (HIV). HIV damages the body's defence system. People who have AIDS die because their body can no longer fight off other serious illnesses.

- People infected with HIV usually go for many years without any sign of disease. They may look and feel perfectly normal and healthy for all of that time. But anybody infected with HIV can infect others.

- AIDS is the late stage of HIV infection It takes an average of 7-10 years to develop – from the time when a person is first infected with HIV. AIDS is not curable, although some medicines have been developed to keep people with AIDS healthier for longer.

- Anyone who suspects that he or she may be infected with HIV should contact a health worker or an AIDS testing centre. It is vital for those who have the virus to learn how to avoid passing it to others, and to receive advice about how to take care of their own health.

HIV can only be passed from one person to another in a limited number of ways:

- By sexual intercourse, during which the semen or vaginal fluid of an infected person passes into the body of another person. HIV can be passed in this way from man to man, man to woman, and woman to man. Worldwide, nine out of ten infections in adults have been passed on through sexual intercourse.

- By the use of unsterilized needles or syringes for injecting drugs.

- By blood transfusions, if the blood used has not been tested for HIV.

- By an infected woman to her unborn child.

● If a mother is infected with HIV, then there is a risk that breastfeeding may give the virus to her baby. But where other diseases and malnutrition are a common cause of death in babies, not breastfeeding is a much greater risk. Without safe water, sterile bottles and teats, and enough milk-powder, bottle-fed babies are much more likely to become ill and malnourished, and to die, than babies who are breastfed. In such conditions, it is safer for the child to be breastfed even if the mother is infected with HIV.

● It is not possible to get HIV from being near to or touching those who are infected with the virus. Hugging, shaking hands, coughing and sneezing will not spread the disease. HIV cannot be transmitted by toilets seats, telephones, plates, glasses, spoons, towels, bed linen, swimming pools, or public baths.

● A person infected with HIV is not a public health danger.

2 | **People who are sure that both they and their partner are uninfected and have no other sex partners are not at risk from AIDS. People who know or suspect that this might not be the case should practise safer sex. This means either sex without intercourse (penetration), or intercourse only when protected by a condom.**

● Mutual fidelity between two uninfected partners protects both people from HIV.

● The more sex partners you have, the greater the risk that one of them will be infected and can infect you. The more partners your partner has, the greater the risk that he or she will be infected and can infect you.

● People who have genital sores, ulcers, or inflammation, or a discharge from the vagina or penis, are at greater risk of becoming infected with HIV and of passing it to others. Prompt treatment for all genital infections is therefore very important.

● Unless you and your partner have sex only with each other, and are sure you are both uninfected, you should reduce your risk of HIV by practising safer sex. Safer sex means kissing, caressing and other kinds of non-penetrative sex (where the penis does not enter the mouth, vagina or anus), or using a condom (a sheath or rubber) every time you have intercourse.

● Even if a condom is used, anal intercourse (in which the penis enters the rectum or back passage) is much more risky than vaginal or oral penetration.

● The only way to avoid any such risk is to abstain from sex.

3 | Any injection with an unsterilized needle or syringe is dangerous.

● A needle or syringe can pick up small amounts of blood from the person being injected. If that person's blood contains HIV, and if the same needle or syringe is used for injecting another person without being sterilized first, then HIV can be injected.

● Those who inject themselves with drugs are therefore particularly at risk from AIDS. So are people who have sex with those who inject drugs.

Drug injecting is in itself dangerous. But because of the additional risk of HIV, those who do inject drugs should never use another person's needle or syringe or allow their own needle or syringe to be used by anyone else.

● National child immunization programmes use needles that are sterilized between each use and are therefore safe. All infants should be taken for a full course of immunization in the first year of life.

● Other injections are often unnecessary, as many useful medicines can be taken by mouth. Where injections are necessary, they should be given only by a trained person using a sterilized needle and syringe.

● Ear-piercing, dental treatment, tattooing, facial marking and acupuncture are not safe if the equipment used is not sterilized. It is also not safe to be shaved by a barber using an unsterilized razor.

4 | Women infected with HIV should think carefully about having a baby – and seek advice. There is a one-in-three chance that their babies will also be born infected with HIV.

● Women with HIV infection have about a 30% chance of giving birth to a baby who will also be infected with HIV. Most babies infected with the virus will die before they are three years old.

● In some countries, HIV tests are available to couples who are concerned that one or both of them might be infected. The results can help them decide whether to have children. Even if only the man is infected, the woman may become infected through sexual intercourse while attempting to conceive, thereby putting herself and her baby at risk.

5 | All parents should tell their children how HIV is spread.

● Apart from protecting yourself and your partner, you can also help to protect your children against HIV by making sure they know the facts about how to avoid getting and spreading the infection.

● Children also need to know the facts about how HIV *does not* spread. They need to be reassured that they run no risk of getting the virus from ordinary social contact with HIV-infected children or adults. Children should be encouraged to be sympathetic towards people who are infected with HIV.

● Everyone can help in the worldwide effort to stop HIV from spreading to the new generation.

OBJECTIVES for children's understanding and action

Children should:

● Understand that AIDS is incurable.

● Understand how HIV is spread and that it can be spread by people who appear to be well.

● Understand that HIV is not spread by normal social contact.

● Understand what decisions they have to make to avoid being infected with HIV.

● Know how to resist sexual pressure from adults, e.g. those in authority, friends of the family.

● Understand that people infected with HIV and AIDS in families and communities need help and friendship from other community members including children.

UNDERSTANDING about AIDS

1. Collecting health information material and using it to find out about HIV and AIDS

(This activity is suitable for children from 10 years old.)

Finding out

Ask the children to collect pamphlets, posters and other information material available in the community that tells about HIV and AIDS and other STDs (sexually transmitted diseases).

Learning about it

Organize the children in groups to look at the materials and to share what they have learnt. They find the answers to three questions: Why is HIV dangerous? How is it spread? How can we avoid getting it?

Checking that we know and understand about it

When children display the posters and the material they have collected, organize a quiz to check that they know the facts about HIV and AIDS, e.g.:

> Ask children to give sentences on what they know about HIV and AIDS. Make a list by writing them on the board. Each group then has a chance to respond to one sentence by saying 'true' or 'false', whichever they think is correct. Another group can challenge if they disagree. They use the pamphlets and posters to decide the right answer.

(See Facts for Life information to check that all information is correct.)

2. Role-play . . . to practise saying 'no'

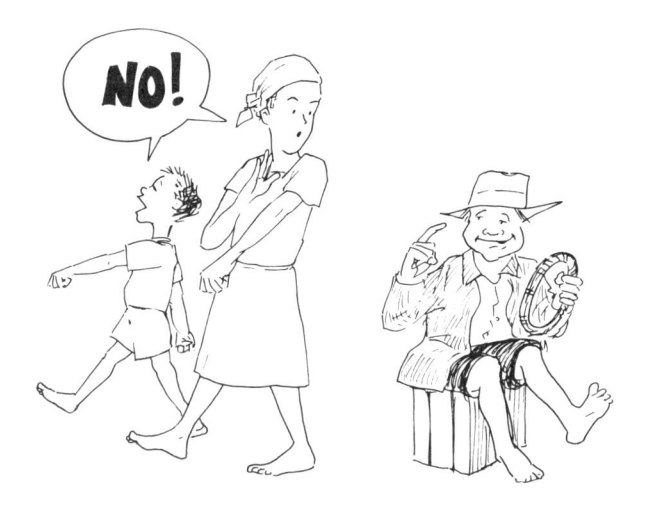

Talk with children about situations when it is sometimes difficult to say 'no'.

List the situations and decide if they involve unsafe health practices.

List the reasons why it is difficult to say 'no' to unsafe health practices – like drinking alcohol, smoking, taking drugs.

Discuss strong ways to say 'no' to people who try to get us to do something we know is an unsafe practice.

Ask children to imagine how people might try to persuade them into an unsafe practice; how would they say 'no' in a way which is polite but firm? For example, when asked to have a cigarette; to drink alcohol; to go somewhere with a stranger; to go somewhere with a person they know but think it is not right to be alone with; to try taking drugs; to have sexual intercourse.

Put the children in groups or pairs and let them choose a situation to practise saying 'no'. In each group, one or two of them are the persuaders and the others are the 'no-sayers'. They act out the situation.

Help them to discuss the role-play:

- How did you feel when you were asked to do the unsafe thing?
- How did you feel when the persuaders would not accept your 'no'?
- In the real situation, what might make you change your mind?

and

- Why did you want to persuade your friend to do the unsafe thing?
- How did you feel when your friend said 'no'?
- What kind of answer would make you stop trying to persuade your friend to do what they did not want to do?

At the end, summarize the importance of saying 'no' to unsafe practices that can lead to getting HIV and AIDS and spreading it.

3. Activities about attitudes to people who have AIDS

Help children to:

• Use pictures, e.g. of someone caring for a friend with AIDS. Ask them to imagine how they would feel in the role of one person in the picture. They can ask questions about what events led to the scene shown and what might happen in the future.

• Create short plays, for example about caring at home for a person with AIDS. They can first act the play for themselves, then each make a simple puppet for their character and perform the play with puppets for the rest of the school or the community.

• Fill in the details of a story, for example about an imaginary school pupil thought to have AIDS. The children divide into groups representing the pupil, other pupils, teachers and parents. Each group separately considers: 'What do I feel?', 'What are the main effects on me?', and 'What do I want to happen?' After 15 minutes the groups reassemble and share their discussions.

CHILDREN'S ACTION

I Can

- Be strong and say 'no' to unsafe practices.
- Help someone who has HIV or AIDS.
- Write a poem about AIDS and read it to the family.
- Collect and share stories from religious books of people caring for the sick.

We Can

- Make a drama about a bad character (HIV). It tries to lead people into unsafe practices. Some, but not all, adults can be persuaded. A group of children have learnt how to avoid it and how to tell other people about the dangers. The HIV character finds that fewer and fewer people will listen to it.

  Perform the play for other children and in the community. (In many countries, such children's performances have been used widely in AIDS campaigns.)

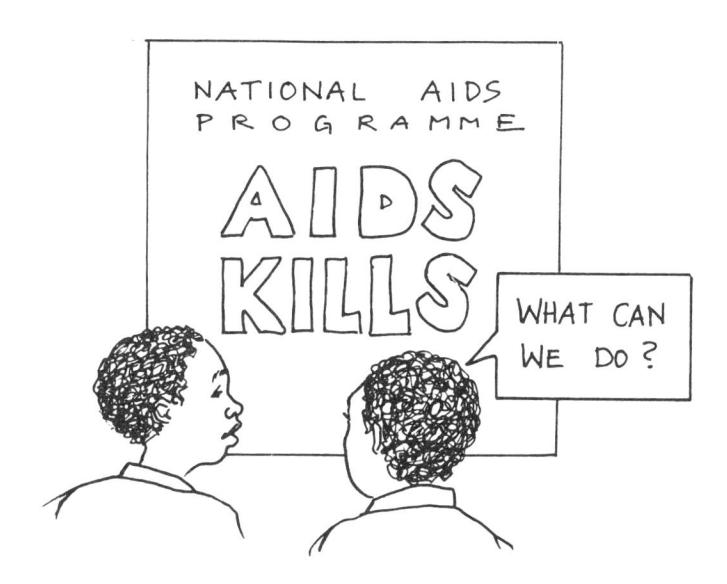

- Make posters with the facts about HIV and AIDS and display them at the school and clinic, and in the neighbourhood.

● Start an anti-AIDS club.

> **How to organize an anti-AIDS club**
> ☐ Find a patron to provide support and funding.
> ☐ Find a place to meet.
> ☐ Ask local health workers or AIDS campaign workers to give talks and advice.
> ☐ Make a plan for regular meetings, and ask other children to join the club.
> ☐ Decide on a membership pledge and rules for all who join.
> ☐ Discuss and plan a series of weekly activities, e.g. visits, talks, drama, performing songs and dances, making posters.

A BASKET OF IDEAS

● Teachers find out about national anti-AIDS programmes. What part can children play in them?

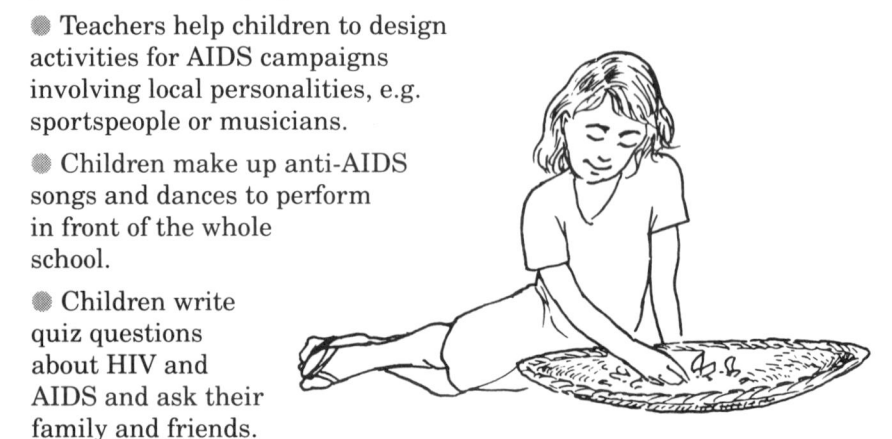

● Teachers help children to design activities for AIDS campaigns involving local personalities, e.g. sportspeople or musicians.

● Children make up anti-AIDS songs and dances to perform in front of the whole school.

● Children write quiz questions about HIV and AIDS and ask their family and friends.

EVALUATION QUESTIONS

Children

- Do I know the main facts about HIV and AIDS and how it is spread?
- Have I explained the facts about HIV and AIDS to another child?

- Am I confident about saying 'no' if I have to?
- Have I helped someone who has HIV or AIDS?

Teachers

- How well do all children remember what does and does not spread HIV?
- Have children demonstrated their knowledge and attitudes about HIV and AIDS, e.g. by writing a story about someone who has AIDS?

Health Workers

- How many local schools and youth groups teach about HIV and AIDS?
- How many schools have organized activities about HIV and AIDS in school-based clubs, e.g. scouts, Red Cross and Red Crescent?

In many countries parents and communities may feel uneasy about transmitting the explicit information in this AIDS section to children. Those who transmit the messages need to be aware of cultural sensitivities when they decide at what age different information is given. They must reflect, however, on the need for children to know these life-preserving facts before they become sexually active and it is too late.

What children need to know and pass on about
Safe Motherhood

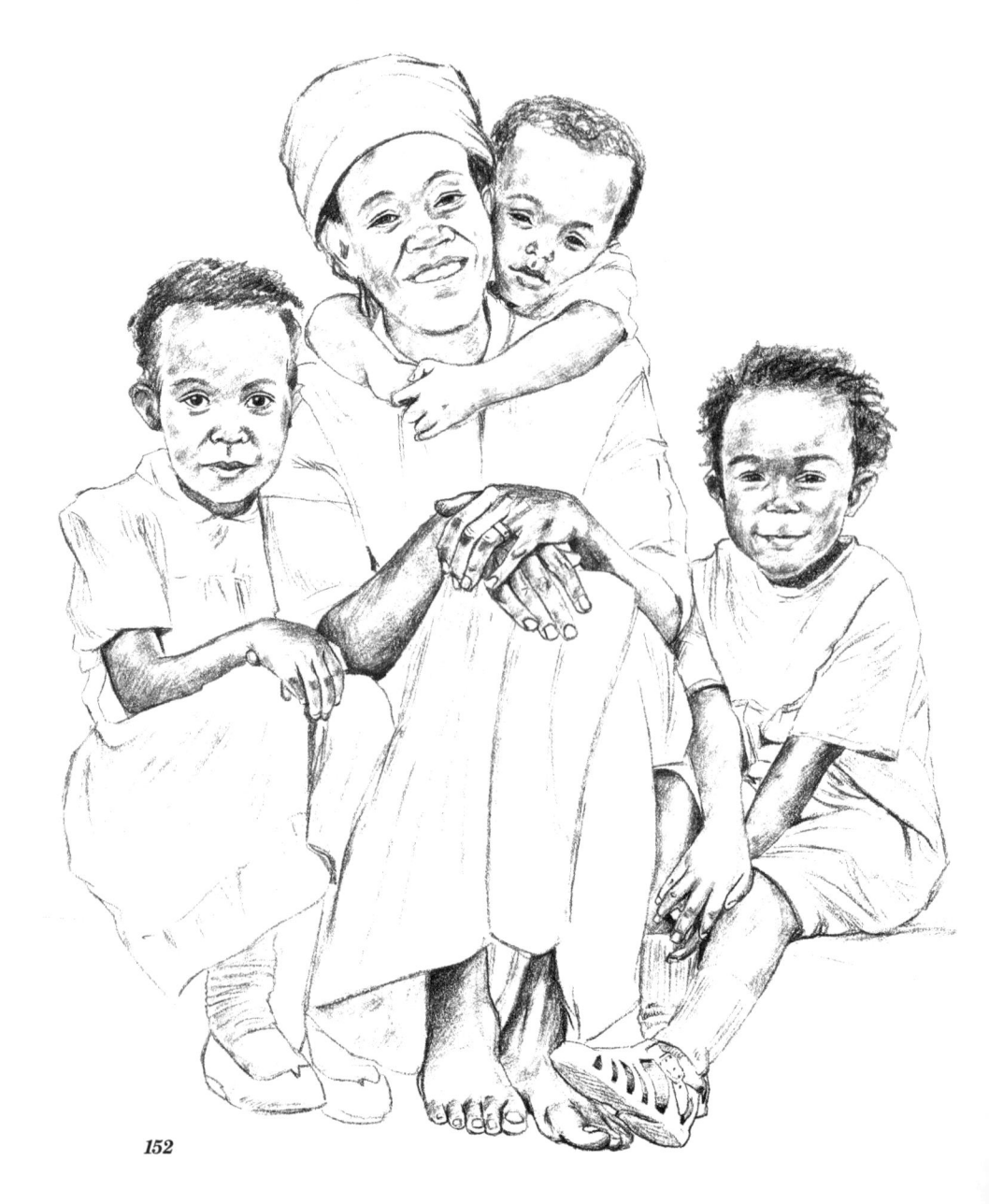

Although the prime messages concerning Timing Births and Safe Motherhood appear to be mainly for adults, children also need to understand them, for two reasons. First, children are future parents and second, there are ways, as family members, that they can help their mothers and fathers to keep babies safe and healthy before birth and after they are born.

In societies where customs persist which can harm the health of mothers (e.g. very early marriage and pregnancy; use of untrained people as birth attendants), the school, together with the health worker, may have a responsibility to transmit correct messages to future parents.

PRIME MESSAGES
and supporting information

Timing births

1 Becoming pregnant before the age of 18, or after the age of 35, increases the health risks for both mother and child.

● Every year over half a million women die from problems linked to pregnancy and childbirth, leaving behind over one million motherless children. Most of these deaths could be prevented by acting on today's knowledge about the importance of planning pregnancies.

All girls should be allowed the time to become women before becoming mothers. In societies where many girls marry at an early age, couples should delay the first pregnancy until at least the age of 18.

● For health reasons alone, no girl should become pregnant before the age of 18. A woman is not physically ready to begin bearing children until she is about 18 years of age. Babies born to women younger than 18 are more likely to be born too early and to weigh too little at birth. The birth itself is likely to be more difficult. Babies born to mothers who are too young are also much more likely to die in the first year of life. The risks to the mother's own health are also greater.

153

● After the age of 35, the health risks of pregnancy and childbirth begin to increase again. If a woman is over the age of 35, and has had four or more previous pregnancies, then another pregnancy is a serious risk to her own health and that of her unborn child.

2 | **The risk of death for young children is increased by about 50% if the space between births is less than two years.**

● For the health of both mothers and children, parents should wait until their youngest child is at least two years old before having another baby.

● Children born too close together do not usually develop as well, physically or mentally, as children born at least two years apart.

● One of the greatest threats to the health and growth of a child under the age of two is the birth of a new baby. Breastfeeding stops too suddenly, and the mother has less time to prepare the special foods a young child needs. Also, she may not be able to give the older child the care and attention he or she needs, especially during illness. As a result, the child often fails to grow and develop properly.

● A mother's body needs two years to recover fully from pregnancy and childbirth. The risk to the mother's health is therefore greater if the next birth follows too closely upon the last. The mother needs to give herself time to get her strength and energy back before she becomes pregnant again.

● If a woman becomes pregnant before she is fully recovered from bearing a previous child, there is a higher chance that her new baby will be born too early and too light in weight. Low-birth-weight babies are less likely to grow well, more likely to fall ill, and four times more likely to die in the first year of life than babies of normal weight.

3 | **Having more than four children increases the health risks of pregnancy and childbirth.**

● After a woman has had four children, further pregnancies bring greater risks to the life and health of both mother and child.
 Especially if the previous births have not been spaced more than two years apart, a woman's body can easily become exhausted by repeated pregnancy, childbirth, breastfeeding, and looking after small children. Further pregnancies usually mean that her own health begins to suffer.

● After four pregnancies, there is an increased risk of serious health problems such as anaemia ('thin blood') and haemorrhage (heavy loss of blood). The risk of giving birth to babies with disabilities, or with low birth weight, also increases after four pregnancies and after the mother reaches the age of 35.

4 | **There are many safe and acceptable ways of avoiding pregnancy. Family planning services can give couples the knowledge and the means to plan when to begin having children, how far apart to have them, and when to stop.**

● Most health clinics can offer different methods of family planning so that all couples can choose a method which is acceptable, safe, convenient, and effective. Couples should ask advice about the most suitable means of family planning from the nearest trained health worker or family planning clinic.

● Family planning is the responsibility of men as well as women. All men should be aware of the health benefits of family planning – and of the different methods now available.

Safe motherhood

5 | **The risks of childbirth can be drastically reduced by going to the nearest health worker for regular check-ups during pregnancy.**

● Many of the dangers of pregnancy and childbirth can be avoided if the mother-to-be goes to a health centre as soon as she believes she is pregnant. A health worker will help ensure a safe birth and a healthy baby by:

- ☐ Checking the progress of the pregnancy so that if problems are likely the woman can be moved to a hospital for the birth.
- ☐ Checking for high blood pressure, which is a danger to both mother and child.
- ☐ Giving tablets to prevent anaemia ('thin blood').
- ☐ Giving the two injections which will protect the mother and her newborn baby against tetanus.
- ☐ Checking that the baby is growing properly.
- ☐ Giving anti-malarial tablets where necessary.
- ☐ Preparing the mother for the experience of childbirth and giving advice on breastfeeding and care of the newborn.

- Advising on where to go or how to get help if problems arise during childbirth.
- Advising on ways of delaying the next pregnancy.

6 — A trained person should assist at every birth.

● A trained birth attendant will know:
- When labour has gone on for too long (more than 12 hours) and a move to hospital is necessary.
- How to keep the birth clean and reduce the risk of infection.
- How to cut the cord cleanly and safely.
- What to do if the baby is being born in the wrong position.
- What to do if too much blood is being lost.
- What to do if the baby does not begin breathing straight away.
- How to help the mother to start breastfeeding immediately after the birth.
- How to dry and keep the baby warm after delivery.
- How to help the mother prevent or postpone another birth.

● If serious problems arise during childbirth, a trained birth attendant will know when medical help is needed and how to get it.

7 — To reduce the dangers of pregnancy and childbirth, all families should know the warning signs.

● With any pregnancy, it is important to ask the advice of a health worker about where the baby should be born and who should attend the birth. If a family knows that a birth is likely to be difficult or risky, it may be possible to have the baby in a hospital or maternity clinic. Or it may be possible to move, temporarily, closer to a clinic or hospital so that the mother is within reach of medical help. The following are the **warning signs to note during pregnancy**:

- Failure to gain weight (at least six kilos should be gained in pregnancy).
- Paleness of inside eyelids (should be red or pink).
- Unusual swelling of legs, arms, or face.

Four signs which mean get help immediately:
- Bleeding from the vagina during pregnancy.

☐ Severe headaches (sign of high blood pressure).

☐ Severe vomiting.

☐ High fever.

● Dangerous problems can arise during the process of giving birth. In at least half of all cases, there are no warning signs in pregnancy. Therefore all couples should know – *in advance* – where the nearest hospital or maternity unit is to be found and how to get there. In case problems arise during labour, the father-to-be should make advance arrangements for moving the mother-to-be to the nearest hospital or maternity unit. In particular, transport should be arranged in case it is needed.

8 | All women need more food during pregnancy. All pregnant women need more rest.

● The husband and family of a pregnant woman should ensure that she has a variety of extra foods every day – starting as soon as pregnancy is confirmed. She should also have more rest than usual during the daytime, especially in the three months before the birth.

● A pregnant woman needs a variety of the best foods available to the family: milk, fruit, vegetables, meat, fish, eggs, pulses, and grains. There is no reason to avoid any of these foods during pregnancy.

● If possible, a woman should be weighed as soon as she knows that she is pregnant. It is important to gain weight every month during pregnancy, and to try to gain a total of 8-10 kilos before the baby is born.

9 | Spacing pregnancies at least two years apart, and avoiding pregnancies below the age of 18 or above the age of 35, drastically reduces the dangers of child-bearing.

● One of the most effective ways of reducing the dangers of pregnancy and childbirth – for both mother and child – is to plan the timing of births. The risks of child-bearing are greatest when the mother-to-be is under 18 or over 35, or has had four or more previous pregnancies, or when there is a gap of less than two years since the last birth.

● Avoiding births by having an unsafe abortion can be very dangerous. Illegal abortions carried out by untrained persons kill between 100,000 and 200,000 women every year.

10 Girls who are healthy and well fed during their own childhood and teenage years have fewer problems in pregnancy and childbirth.

● Safe and successful child-bearing depends most of all on the health and readiness of the mother-to-be. So special attention should be paid to the health, feeding, and education of adolescent girls. The first pregnancy should wait until at least the age of 18.

11 If a woman who is pregnant smokes, or takes alcohol or drugs, her child may be damaged in the womb.

● A pregnant woman can damage her unborn child by smoking tobacco, drinking alcohol, and using narcotic drugs. It is particularly important not to take medicines during pregnancy unless they are absolutely necessary and prescribed by a trained health worker.

N.B. Some of the supporting information included in *Facts for Life* has been omitted or shortened.

OBJECTIVES for children's understanding and action

Children should:

● Understand that a pregnant woman needs to have rest, and a sufficient and balanced diet; and should avoid harmful drugs, alcohol and smoking.

● Understand that a pregnant woman needs to go to the nearest health worker for regular check-ups and advice; and also needs to be immunized against tetanus.

● Understand that a trained attendant needs to be present at every birth. The attendant will know when medical help is needed and how to get it.

● Understand that the health of both mother and children can suffer when the space between births is too short.

● Know how to help mothers who are pregnant, by helping in the home and with younger children.

UNDERSTANDING about safe motherhood

1. Discussion and role-play based on a picture

Show a picture of a mother and four children (aged six months, two years, three-and-a-half years, and five years).

Discuss:

- What does mother have to do for each of these children?
- What can each of these children do on their own?
- What can they do to help each other?
- Who helps mother?
- Who helps the children?
- What happens if nobody helps mother?
- What happens if mother gets sick, or if more than one child gets sick at the same time?

Role-play:

- Children take the roles of the mother and each of the four small children, including the baby.
- The role-play should explore possible problems and benefits, from each one's point of view, e.g. 'My mother gets very tired and cannot spend much time with me'; 'I am jealous of the baby'; 'We can all play together'.

2. A demonstration and discussion ... what happens when plants (food plants or trees) grow too close together?

Children:

- Grow seeds in two pots, or plots; one with seeds planted very close together, another with seeds properly spaced.
- Visit a farm, or a wood, before plants are thinned.
- Look at a picture:

TOO CLOSE TOGETHER   ENOUGH SPACE BETWEEN THEM

They discuss:

- In what way do these examples relate to child-spacing?
- In what way are they different?

3. A visit from the health worker ... protecting the unborn child

The health worker explains to the children how a baby grows in the womb and why it can be damaged if the mother drinks alcohol or takes harmful drugs, or the mother or father smoke.

Are there are any posters or pamphlets on this theme? If so, children collect, display and make their own copies.

4. A demonstration ... the shortest and most dangerous journey

If it is culturally acceptable, the health worker and teacher can demonstrate, using diagrams (or, better still, models*) how a baby makes the shortest and most dangerous journey of its life, i.e. from the womb to the world.

This activity helps children to understand why it is necessary for a trained person to assist at birth.

CHILDREN'S ACTION

I Can

- Help my mother or aunt when she is pregnant, so that she has time to rest.
- Tell my older sisters and aunts about anti-tetanus injections.

We Can

- Put on a play, *'Who knows best?'*, comparing nutrition before and after pregnancy in two families.
- Help look after younger children when mothers go for health checks during pregnancy.

BASKET OF IDEAS

- Children draw a map to show where trained birth attendants live.
- Children write a story about early marriage and pregnancy: a girl marries and has a baby while she is still very young and at school. What happens?

---

*Good models that can be assembled by the teacher are available, e.g. from Teaching-aids At Low Cost (address on page 183).

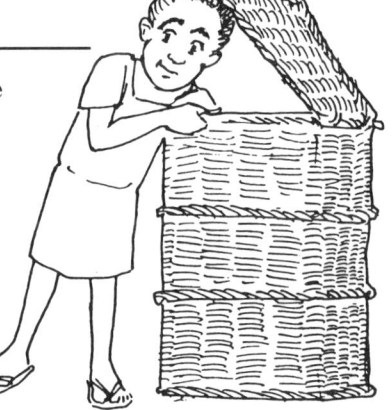

EVALUATION QUESTIONS

Children
- Can we list the problems of too small birth intervals?
- Can we say what we have done to help mother when she is pregnant?

Teachers
- Can children list what a mother needs to have, and to avoid, to keep a baby healthy in the womb? Can they list what fathers need to do?
- What are parents' reactions to children learning about birth spacing and safe motherhood? What have we done to convince them that this knowledge is acceptable and important for children?

Health Workers
- Have schools taught their children simple facts about safe motherhood? Have we been involved?

What children need to know and pass on about
Accidents

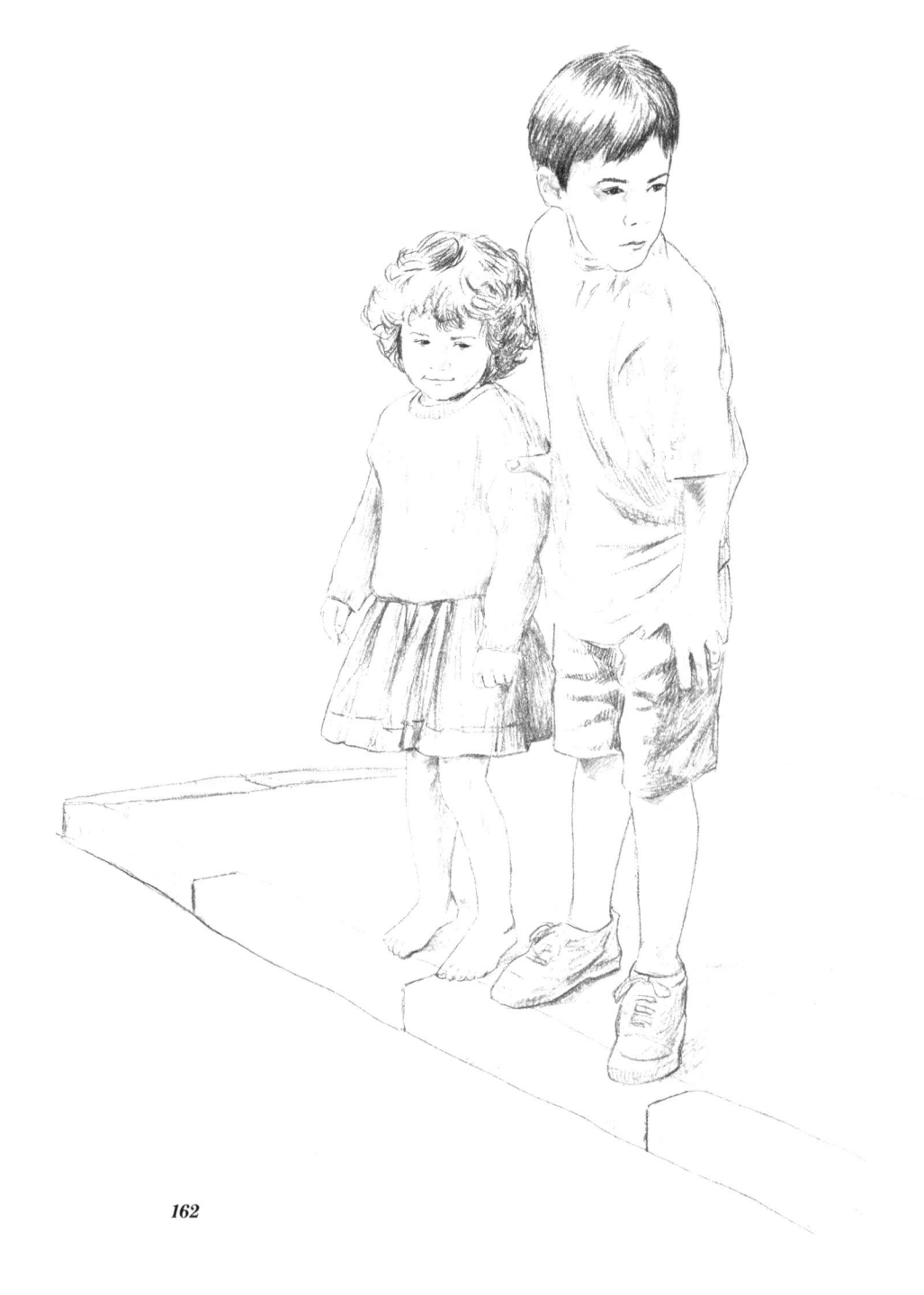

Babies and young children are at risk in and around the home, and on the roads. Many die. Many are seriously injured. Yet nearly all of these accidents can be prevented.

Children have an important role in helping to prevent accidents to each other, and in helping to make adults aware of the dangers children face as a result of careless behaviour.

PRIME MESSAGES
and supporting information

1 Children under four years old are particularly at risk in the home. This is where most deaths and serious accidents occur. Almost all can be prevented.

- The main causes of accidents for little children are:
  - Burns from cooking pots, lamps and electrical equipment, hot food, boiling water, steam and hot fat (scalds); and strong acids or corrosives (like battery acid) which damage the skin.
  - Cuts from broken glass, rusty pins, rough wood or sharp knives and axes.
  - Obstruction (prevention) of breathing from choking on small objects like coins, buttons and nuts.
  - Poisonous plants and fruit.
  - Internal (inside) bleeding from swallowing sharp objects.
  - Electric shock from touching a broken electrical appliance or electrical wire. Electrical wires and connections should be checked regularly. Bare wires are particularly dangerous.

2 Families need to take special care to make their home environment safe and to watch little children to prevent them from unsafe behaviour. Remember that houses are not designed for children, particularly children under two. Try always to look at safety at home with a young child in mind.

DANGER FROM BURNS

● The kitchen is the most dangerous place for children, and burns and scalds the most common causes of death and serious accidents. Take particular care. There are many ways to prevent burns at home:

- ☐ Watch babies and young children very carefully. Do not let them go near the fire.
- ☐ Raise the family cooking stove, or make an open cooking fire on a raised mound of clay instead of directly on the ground.
- ☐ Be very careful that the handles of cooking pots are out of reach of babies and turned so that they are not easily knocked over.
- ☐ Put petrol, petrol lamps and matches out of reach of small children.

DANGER FROM POISON

● Young children are often injured or even killed when they eat or drink dangerous things.

● Never put dangerous products (e.g. bleach, plant poison, paraffin [kerosene], petrol or pesticides) in a soft drink bottle. Children can drink them by mistake.

● Keep all medicines and poisons out of reach, and out of sight, of children. Lock medicines and poisons in a cupboard or trunk, or put them on a high shelf. Label all poisons and medicines carefully. Medicines are particularly dangerous because little children often eat tablets thinking they are sweets.

● Teach young children not to drink out of strange bottles or eat strange fruits and plants which may not be safe.

DANGER FROM SHARP THINGS

● Many cuts can be easily prevented:

- ☐ Keep the floor clean of broken glass and nails. Get rid of nails or splinters of wood which stick out.
- ☐ Keep sharp knives and razors out of the reach of young children.

DANGER FROM FALLS

● Discourage little children from climbing into unsafe places.

● Where there are windows, be very careful. Children can fall from them and can also be cut if they break the glass.

3 Places where children often play should be made as safe as possible. All glass bottles should be banned. Older children must learn to take responsibility for the safety of younger ones at play.

● Children above four years are particularly at risk outside the home as they begin to explore their environment.

● Encourage children to avoid dangerous places in the neighbourhood where there may be machinery, animals, snakes, glass or sharp metal.

● Make wells safe so that children cannot fall in.

● Teach children to teach each other to play safely, in particular to avoid:
- Climbing in dead trees.
- Swimming in swift-flowing rivers, and swimming alone.
- Throwing stones and other sharp things.

● Where there is a playground, check carefully and regularly:
- That the equipment is safe and not rotten.
- That children of the right age are using the equipment.
- That little children are supervised.

4 Chilren under five years old are particularly at risk on the roads. They should be watched and taught appropriate safety behaviour as soon as they can walk.

● Little children do not think before they run out into the road. They cannot estimate how fast vehicles are travelling, and cannot tell by listening where a vehicle is coming from.

● Families need to watch little children carefully, and teach them when they are young, always to:
- Stop at the road side.
- Hold the hand of an older person when crossing the road.

● Older children should be taught to:
- Choose safe places to cross.
- Look both ways and listen every time they cross.

● Older children must always take responsibility for younger ones.

● Little children should be discouraged from playing with balls near the roadside.

165

● Children who ride bicycles need to be given special training.

5 | All families need to know simple first aid – particularly that related to burns, cuts and wounds, and swallowing poisons and other objects. Many common practices are dangerous to health.

FIRST AID FOR WOUNDS AND CUTS

● If the wound is not serious:
- Wash the wound with very clean (or boiled) water and soap.
- Dry the skin around the wound.
- Cover the wound and the skin around it with a very clean pad of cloth (not cotton wool or any fluffy material) and bandage it in place.
- Wash the wound and put on a clean bandage every day.

● If the wound is serious:
- If there is a lot of bleeding, press firmly against the wound (or near to it if there is something stuck in it). Use your hand if you have no cloth.
- Put a bandage on the wound and take the person to the health worker.
- If the person has not been recently immunized against tetanus, tell the health worker, who should begin the immunization course immediately.

REMEMBER:

● Do not put any plant or animal matter on the wound.

FIRST AID FOR BURNS

● Remove the person from the source of the heat. If a person's clothing is on fire, wrap them in a blanket or roll them on the ground to put out the fire.

● **Cool the burnt area immediately** using lots of cold, clean water. It may take up to half an hour to cool the burnt area. If the burn is very large, put the person into a bath of cold water.

● **For small burns** (less than the size of a large coin or stamp):
- Keep the burnt area clean and dry, and protect it with a loose bandage. If the burn is bigger than a large coin, show it to a health worker.

● **For large (serious) burns:**
  □ Cover the burnt area with a dry and very clean piece of cloth, and get medical help immediately.

REMEMBER:

● Do not break the blisters.

● Do not remove any clothing which is sticking to the burnt area.

● Do not put grease, oil or herbs on the burn.

FIRST AID FOR POISON

● Do not try to make the person vomit.

● Seek the help of a health worker immediately.

● Try to find out what the poison was and take it with you to the health worker.

N.B. The prime messages and supporting information in this section do not appear in *Facts for Life*. This section has been specially prepared for *Children for Health*.

OBJECTIVES for children's understanding and action

Children should:

● Understand the causes of common accidents in the home and how they can be prevented.

● Understand their responsibility, alongside adults, to watch over others, particularly younger children, to prevent unsafe behaviour.

● Know and practise road safety rules for themselves and with friends.

● Know how to make their neighbourhood safe and choose safe places to play.

● Know and practise simple first aid for burns, cuts and wounds. Know which common practices are useful.

UNDERSTANDING about accidents

1. A survey and discussion ... accidents in our families

• Children record accidents that have happened to members of their families. They make three lists or graphs of accidents which happened at home, on the road, and out-of-doors; and decide which kind of accidents happen most often in the community.

Why do children think these accidents happen? If they can discover why they happen, they can also find out how to **prevent them from happening so often**.

• Children discuss which accidents are most common for children at different ages (and why) – under two years, from two to six years, after six years.

2. Role-play based on pictures

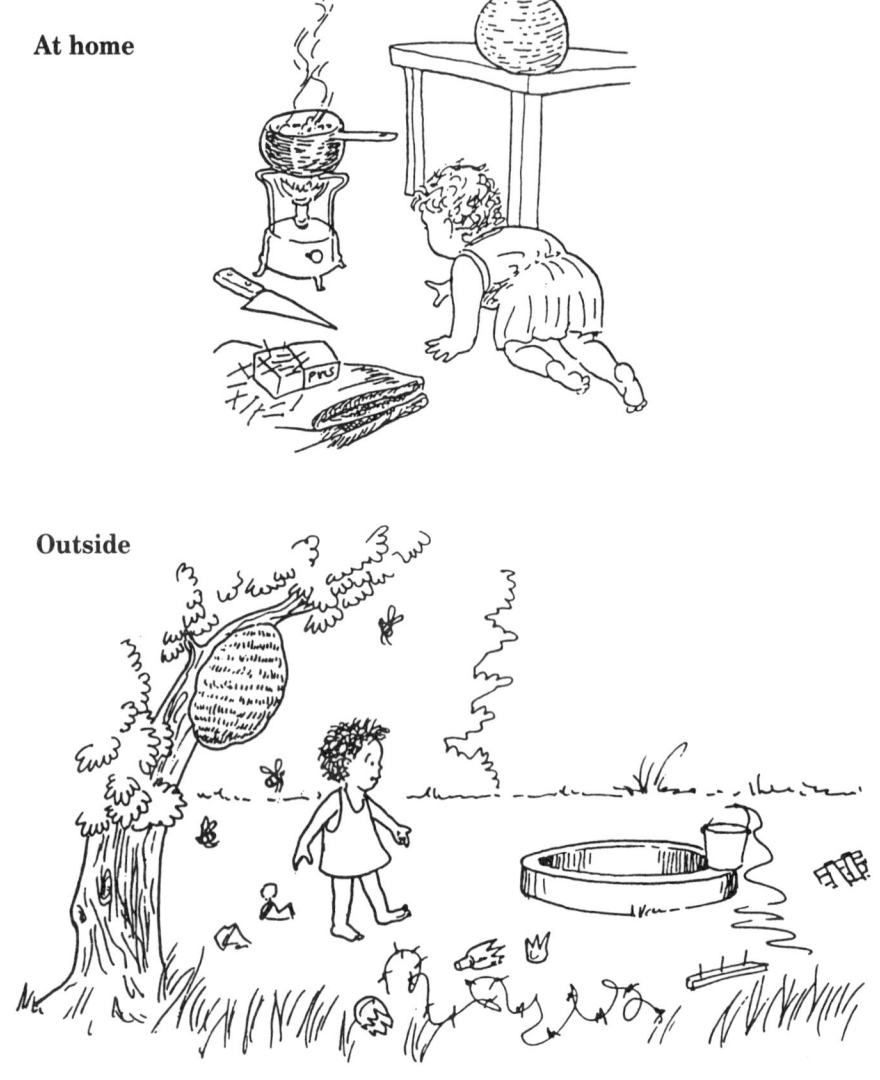

At home

Outside

• Discussion ... what is it like to be a baby or young child?

- Children make a 'dangerous home' and a 'safe home' in the classroom. They crawl among the hazards.

3. First aid ... practising what to do

Children watch a demonstration and then practise in pairs how they would act in situations where simple first aid is needed, e.g. a burn on a child's arm; a cut on a child's foot.

4. Drawing and discussion about road accidents

Draw some different road situations on the board:

☐ A school on a wide straight road with heavy lorry traffic.

☐ A bend on the road with trees and bushes alongside.

☐ A playground on a street with many parked cars.

Make the drawings very simple.

Children look at the drawings and suggest where and why accidents can happen, and what they should do to prevent them:

☐ If they are children crossing the road.

☐ If they were adult road users.

5. Using the school playground to teach children about road safety

Draw 'roadways' on the ground and ask children to practise crossing the road. Make it more interesting by creating some dangerous situations.

Some children act as fast cars, overloaded lorries, bushes, parked vehicles, policemen, or careless drivers.

Back in the classroom, children in pairs or groups make lists of rules for crossing the road safely and present them to the class. Which set of rules is the clearest and most useful?

CHILDREN'S ACTION

I Can

● Survey my own home. What dangers are there? What does my family do to protect babies and small children from these dangers? What more could I do? What could I suggest to my family?

● Watch over younger children at home, on the roads, and on the way to school.

● Make up a song about road safety to a popular tune, and teach it to little ones.

● Practise road safety as a pedestrian and a cyclist.

We Can

● Make up, illustrate and display our own safety codes for home and school, e.g. a big sister's/brother's code for looking after little ones; a cyclist's code. Different groups can make their own codes on the same theme, then discuss and combine them to make a final version.

● Organize a safety campaign based on the school. (Do not try to cover everything. Find out the most common causes of accidents and concentrate on those, one at a time.) The campaign should include practical actions to make the school safe.

● Learn, and teach each other simple first aid.

● Make first aid kits for school and home.

A basic first aid kit

12 triangular bandages*

Antiseptic cream

Safety pins

Cotton wool

A torch

Sticking plasters

A thermometer

*each made from a square metre of clean cloth cut in half

● Establish a first aid post at school.

BASKET OF IDEAS

● Children make a hazard map of their local area and identify the danger spots.

● Children hold a traffic survey outside school and watch for dangerous behaviour.

● The teacher invites a policeman to visit the school and talk to children about accidents.

● Children write and perform plays and puppet shows about accidents and what can be done to reduce them.

● The school organizes a poster competition on a particular theme, e.g. dangers in the kitchen. Children make up catchy slogans.

EVALUATION QUESTIONS

Children

- What changes have we and our families made in our homes to make them safer?
- What changes have we made in our school to make it safer?
- What changes have we helped to make in our neighbourhood to make it safer?
- Do we watch little children to protect them from danger?
- Do we help younger children to cross the road?
- Have we taught them our safety rules?
- Are we following our safety rules when we walk and cross the road? if we ride a bicycle?

Teachers

- Have the children carried out a safety campaign?
- Do they know simple first aid for cuts, wounds and burns?
- Have they made first aid boxes for home and classroom?
- Are they used and re-stocked?

Health Workers

- Is there any change in the number of accidents since the safety campaign?
- Are people in the area more aware of correct, simple first aid?
- Are adults more aware of the consequences of careless and dangerous practices, and have they changed their behaviour, e.g. putting medicines out of reach; encouraging authorities to build road humps?

What children need to know and pass on about
Food for the Family

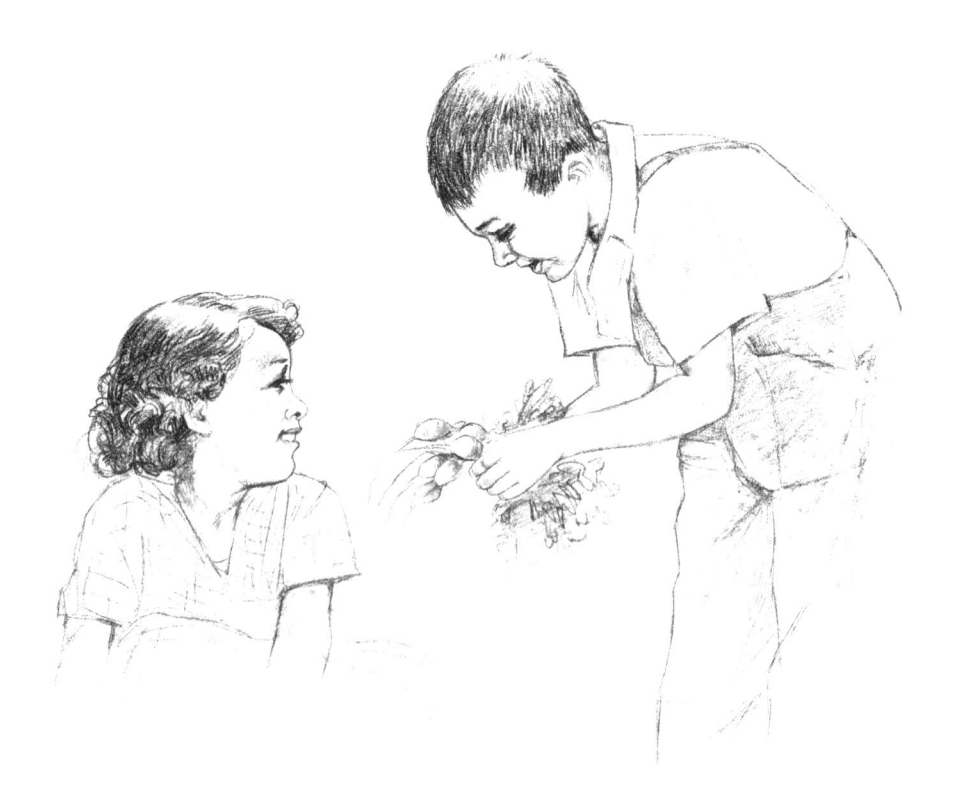

The radishes we grew together

Good nutrition in childhood contributes to both physical and mental growth. Although children, and adults, may not have control of the amount of food available, and when it can be eaten, it is vital to provide the best possible nutrition from what is available. In order to do this, co-operation will be necessary from the whole family, most especially fathers.

PRIME MESSAGES
and supporting information

1 Children need food for their minds as well as their bodies. Good food in the first years increases potential for doing well in school and living a successful and happy life.

- Energy food such as oils, fats and sugar, and food cooked with these, is important for young children. They need energy to run and play. Play is an important part of the learning process.
- In many parts of the world, children are now growing taller than their parents. This is due to better feeding early in their lives.
- Children also grow rapidly during puberty. Good food during this period will help children become healthy mothers and fathers when they are adults.

2 All children need access to the best food available in the family; girls as well as boys, children as well as adults.

- In many cultures, customs suggest to mothers that they should give their husbands and boys more, and the best, food. As a result the difference in size between men and women is greater than it should be.
- Girls who are well fed will do better at school and be more successful in bringing up children. For the best pregnancy, a woman needs to eat well but also to have eaten well as a child.
- Traditional beliefs which suggest that some food, for example eggs and fish, should not be eaten by girls, are being questioned in many countries.
- Parents should understand that even small children need half as much food as their fathers and need varied foods which contain proteins and vitamins.
- In cultures where children share the family meal, mealtimes are seen as a time when adults can share ideas and experience with their children and can pass on their moral and ethical values. Children need to be encouraged to talk about their own activities (e.g. in school) and adults to listen to these.

> **3** All children need to be given the opportunity, and encouraged, to eat frequently. They need a wide variety of available food to help their growth.

● Growing children need continual supplies of energy food to maintain their growth. Therefore it is essential for them to eat often. Social pressures, and those of modern life, often prevent them from doing so.

● Children often suffer from:
- Missing early morning meals because adults go early to work or children go early to school.
- Leaving long gaps between meals in the middle of the day.
- Eating main meals late in the evening when they are too tired to eat properly.

● Parents should do their utmost to ensure that their children do not suffer as a result of infrequent or irregular meals.

● A wide variety of food will ensure that children receive vitamins and minerals as well as the energy and protein needed for activity and growth. These foods include:
- Staple foods, e.g. millet or rice.
- Energy-rich foods, e.g. red palm oil, sunflower oil, margarine, sugar.
- Body-building foods, e.g. beans, peas, lentils, eggs, fish, meat.
- Protective foods, e.g. carrots, oranges, green vegetables.

Many foods, e.g. milk and avocado, fall into more than one of these categories.

> **4** Wherever possible, families need to grow at least some of their own food. Orange or yellow fruits and vegetables, and dark green leafy vegetables, are easy to grow and necessary to provide vitamins which protect the body from illness.

● Orange or yellow fruits and vegetables, and dark green leafy vegetables, are important sources of vitamin A. If people do not have enough vitamin A their resistance to diseases is lowered and they are more likely to be ill and even to die. Severe lack of vitamin A can cause eye problems and even blindness.

● Fruit and vegetables can be grown even in small gardens or in tins or pots. The whole family, including the children, can thus be encouraged to contribute to their own diet, and children can learn skills which they can use as adults.

● Sharing knowledge and skills about growing food, e.g. between older and younger children, between grandparents and children, helps families to live happily and effectively together.

● Some foods, such as fruit, leaves of certain trees, and spinach, have always been collected and eaten. Families can learn to recognize and cook what is available.

> **5** Soil is a resource that cannot be replaced. With more people in the world there is a greater need to make better use of it. Families should preserve and enrich their soil for themselves and their descendants.

● Families must protect their soil from being washed away or blown away. This happens particularly when:

- There is overgrazing.
- The land is not carefully protected, e.g. through contour planting and ridging, and good drainage for water.
- Too many trees are cut down.

● Soil can be enriched by wise choice of crops, and by good use of compost and, where appropriate, animal and human waste.

● Tree planting needs to be encouraged but trees need to be planted in the right places and well tended.

● All families need to become aware of ways of protecting and enriching their soil.

N.B. The prime messages and supporting information in this section do not appear in *Facts For Life*. This section has been specially prepared for *Children for Health*.

OBJECTIVES for children's understanding and action

Children should:

● Understand that different types of food contribute to energy, body-building and protection against disease.

● Understand that all children, girls as well as boys, need good food to promote their physical and mental growth.

● Understand that even small children need half as much food as their fathers. They need to eat often throughout the day, particularly energy-rich foods.

● Understand that orange or yellow fruits and vegetables and dark green leafy vegetables can help to prevent illness; and know how to tend them.

● Understand the need to conserve soil and know how to enrich it and protect it from erosion.

UNDERSTANDING about food for the family

1. A discussion about food ... good food at good prices

Children discuss what foods they usually eat, and how these foods contribute to their health.

Based on their new knowledge (*see pages 173-175*), are there any improvements which could be made in their diets without increasing the costs of food?

2. An eating timetable

Make a simple timetable. Select certain children and ask them to fill in what they ate and when.

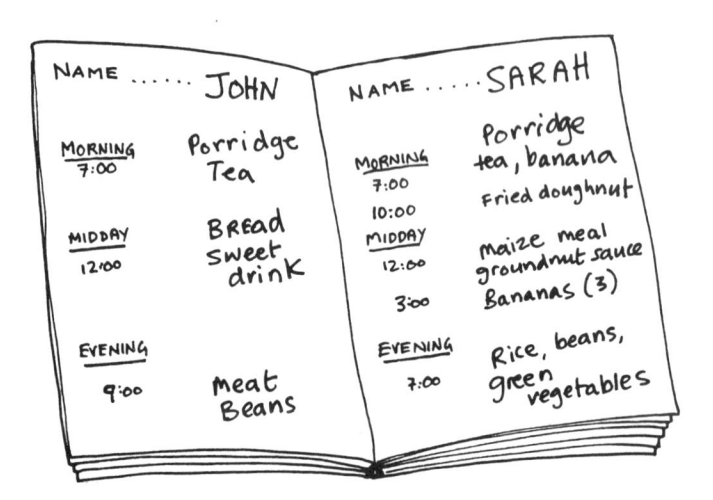

```
NAME ..... JOHN                NAME ..... SARAH

MORNING    Porridge             MORNING    Porridge
 7:00      Tea                   7:00      tea, banana
                                10:00      Fried doughnut
MIDDAY     Bread                MIDDAY     maize meal
12:00      sweet                12:00      groundnut sauce
           drink                 3:00      Bananas (3)

EVENING                         EVENING    Rice, beans,
 9:00      meat                  7:00      green vegetables
           Beans
```

It is important that children who come from the same income group are chosen. (Note that John's food may even cost more than Sarah's but his diet is not as nutritious.)

Make another timetable for children's younger brothers and sisters. (Five or six entries may be needed, rather than just three or four.)

Children discuss in pairs, groups or as a class:

- Did we eat enough at the right time?
- Do our younger brothers and sisters eat often enough?

This is followed up with 'why' and 'what' questions:

- Why do children not have breakfast?
- Why do we eat very late?
- Why do we eat only twice or three times a day?
- What can be done so that children eat more food, more often?

3. A visit to the market ... food value for money

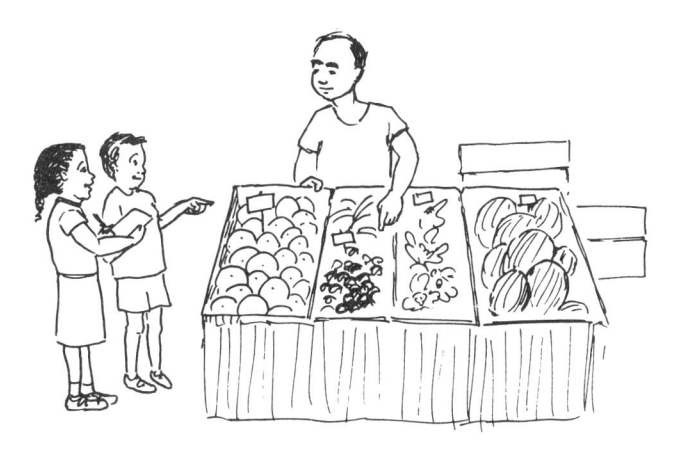

Children visit the local market to find out the cost of food for all the family's meals during one day, and discuss how healthy and appetizing meals can be provided within the family's budget.

4. Learning from a story ... the importance of vitamin A

Tell stories to help children understand that eating orange and yellow fruits and vegetables and dark green leafy vegetables is important for good eyesight and protection against disease.

Stories featuring animals that talk and act as humans are popular in many societies and often a particular characteristic (e.g. wisdom, foolishness) is associated with each animal. Such stories can readily be used to pass on health messages, as the following example shows.

How Hyena tricked Hare

Hyena is miserable. He can no longer see in the dark. He feels weak. The other animals laugh at him, none louder than Hare. Fat and healthy from eating carrots and greens, Hare teases Hyena without mercy, keeping just out of reach. 'Old chicken-eyes,' Hare calls him. In despair, Hyena consults Dr Guinea Fowl who tells him to eat fruit and vegetables. Gradually Hyena's sight and strength come back but he does not tell Hare. Every night Hare continues to tease Hyena. Every night Hyena seems blinder; he even begins to wear dark glasses and use a white stick. Every night Hare gets closer, until one night he gets too close. Hyena pounces. He has his revenge!

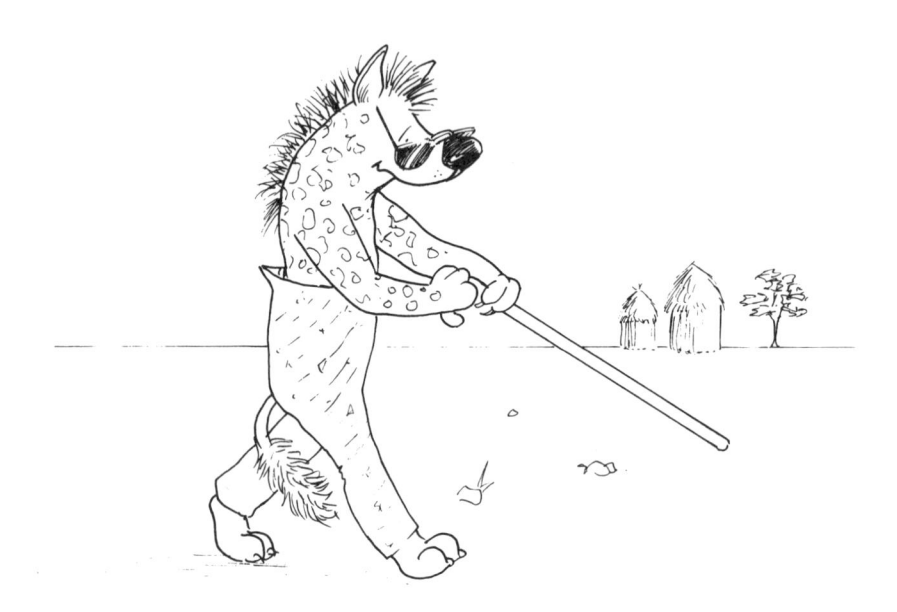

(For ideas about developing stories with children, and follow-up activities, see the section on Immunization.)

5. An experiment and observation ... how do we care for our soil?

- Discuss with the children:
    - Is all soil suitable for growing food?
    - Why is it important to look after the soil on the top? How can we increase it and make it rich?
    - How can the soil be lost?
    - When it is lost, can it be replaced?
    - If it is lost, how could that affect our health?
- In the rainy season, children take some containers and collect samples of run-off water. Is it clear or muddy? Muddy water means

that soil is being washed downstream and lost for farming. Why are the plant roots not holding the water in the soil?

• Children look at farming on hills. Are the rows of plants arranged around the hill (contour planting)? Are there terraces to reduce the amount of soil being washed away?

As a result of the observation, discuss how soil could be preserved better.

CHILDREN'S ACTION

I Can

● Help mother give plenty of small meals to younger brothers and sisters.

● Eat more fruit and green leafy vegetables, if they are available.

● Collect edible wild fruit, nuts and leaves (make sure you know which ones are safe and good to eat).

We Can

● Help to grow fruit and vegetables in a school garden, or agree to have a home plot, and report back to school about what we are growing and doing with the produce.

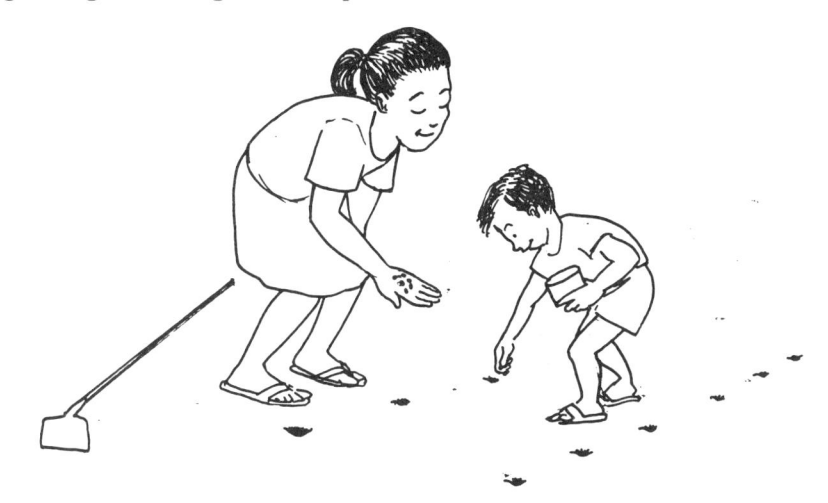

☐ Before starting, discuss practical points. Is it possible to have a vegetable garden at school? Is there enough land, and water? Is fencing needed to keep animals out? Can a crop be grown within one term? Is there a danger of theft?

☐ For some schools it may be better to plant fruit trees in the compound, e.g. pawpaw, mango, orange, banana, avocado, or whatever grows well. The trees need to be protected from goats and cattle when young. Each class could plant and 'adopt' one tree, watering it with hand-washing water. Later, the trees will provide shade as well as fruit.

- ☐ If a vegetable garden is likely to be successful, grow spinach, carrots and other plants rich in vitamin A. Seeds can be planted at home. A small prize, e.g. for the largest carrot, will provide encouragement.

● Make and display posters about foods with vitamin A protecting us from disease.

● Make compost at home and at school to enrich the soil.

● Plant trees and tend them, to prevent soil erosion on slopes.

● Persuade the school food-sellers to stock healthy snacks and drinks, and follow the rules of hygiene.

BASKET OF IDEAS

● Children discuss what foods are eaten at festivals, and why.

● Children survey school food-sellers – which ones sell healthy and clean food?

● Children put on puppet plays to show the importance of vitamin A. Plays can feature animals or people who cannot see well in the dark and show how eating orange or yellow fruits and vegetables, and dark green leafy vegetables, can help them see better. (Remember that vitamin A also improves general health and resistance to disease.)

● Children make and sell healthy snacks to friends.

● Children keep animals for food – fish, rabbits, ducks, chickens and pigs, etc. all provide good food.

● Children ask older people about edible wild plants. They make a display of these plants in class.

● Children hold a cookery demonstration, e.g. new ways to prepare staple foods.

● The teacher asks the local agricultural officer or farmer to advise and help children to make a compost pit, and tell them about mulching.

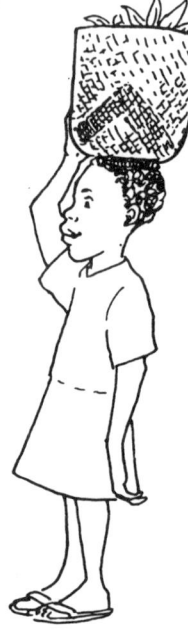

EVALUATION QUESTIONS

Children

- Are we trying to eat more of the right kind of food, e.g. more vegetables?
- Are younger brothers and sisters eating often enough?
- Are we eating often enough (e.g. do we eat before we start school)?
- Do we know ways to conserve soil (especially from erosion)?
- Have we watered and protected the vegetables and trees we planted?
- Are they growing?

Teachers

- Do children know which foods promote growth, energy and health?
- Do they know that orange and yellow fruits and vegetables and dark green leafy vegetables help to provide vitamin A, and why this is important for health?
- Do they understand the idea of 'food value for money in the market'?
- Is school routine organized so that children have time to eat snacks before starting, and during, the school day?
- Are the fruit trees and/or vegetables planted in the school compound well cared for? Will they provide food?
- Are children enthusiastic about planting and watering them? Do they work together?

Agricultural Workers

- Are there any changes in the variety of vegetables and fruit people are growing round their homes? Have the children suggested ideas to their parents?

Some Useful Resources

Books in English

Bonati, G and Hawes, H (eds) (1992). *Child-to-Child: A Resource Book*. London: Child-to-Child Trust.

Feuerstein, M T (1986). *Partners in Evaluation*. London: Macmillan.

Gibbs, W and Mutunga, P (1991). *Health into Mathematics*. Harlow: Longman.

King, M, King, F and Martodipoero, S (1978). *Primary Child Care. Book One*. Oxford: Oxford University Press.

Morley, D and Lovel, H (1986). *My Name is Today*. London: Macmillan.

Savage King, F and Burgess, A (1992). *Nutrition for Developing Countries*. Oxford: ELBS with Oxford University Press.

Werner, D (1993). *Where There is No Doctor*. London: Macmillan.

Werner, D (1987). *Disabled Village Children*. Palo Alto, California: Hesperian Foundation.

Werner, D and Bower, B (1982). *Helping Health Workers Learn*. Palo Alto, California: Hesperian Foundation.

Young, B and Durston, S (1987). *Primary Health Education*. Harlow: Longman.

The above books are available from bookshops or from Teaching-aids At Low Cost (TALC) at the address on page 183.

Story Books for Children in English

Child-to-Child Readers (Harlow: Longman) available from bookshops or TALC:

Easy level 1	Dirty Water
	Good Food
	Accidents
	Not Just a Cold
Level 2	A Simple Cure
	Teaching Thomas
	Down with Fever
	Diseases Defeated
	Flies
	I Can Do It Too
Level 3	Deadly Habits

Adaptations of English story books and parallel series are available:
In Arabic from the Arab Resource Collective.
In Hindi and English from the Voluntary Health Association of India.
In French from L'Enfant pour l'Enfant.
In Spanish from TALC.

Where to Obtain Books and Other Resources

African Medical and Research Foundation (AMREF), Wilson Airport, PO Box 30125, Nairobi, Kenya.
AMREF undertakes health-related materials production and distribution, as well as training and research, mostly in East Africa.

Arab Resource Collective Ltd (ARC), PO Box 7380, Nicosia, Cyprus.
ARC produces, publishes and distributes Arabic-language books and teaching-aids for use in community health and development projects in the Arab world. ARC resources are also available from distributors in Bahrein, Egypt, Jordan, Lebanon, Syria, West Bank and Yemen; details from ARC.

L'Enfant pour l'Enfant, Institut Santé et Développement, 15 rue de l'Ecole de Médecine, 75270 Paris, France.
L'Enfant pour l'Enfant produces materials in French to promote the Child-to-Child approach, assists in implementation in Francophone countries and acts as a resource centre.

Teaching-aids At Low Cost (TALC), PO Box 49, St Albans, Herts AL1 4AX, United Kingdom.
TALC distributes low-cost health books, slides, other teaching-aids and equipment all over the world by mail order. Most titles in English; some also in other languages.

Voluntary Health Association of India (VHAI), Tong Swasthya Bhavan, 40 Institutional Area, South of IIT, New Delhi 110 016, India.
VHAI publishes and distributes books, slides and films in Hindi and English, and provides training and information to grass-roots organizations working in health and community development. State Voluntary Health Associations publish and distribute materials in Indian regional languages; details from VHAI.